Coping with Genetic Disorders offers a storehouse of information and direction for every clergyperson who prepares couples for marriage and for clergy who counsel families reacting to the birth of a child with a genetic disorder. Fletcher clearly describes the choices that face parents, physicians, and counselors at every stage; he points the way for the clergyperson to become "faithful companion" to persons in such crises without being intellectually dishonest or losing the integrity of his or her religious tradition.

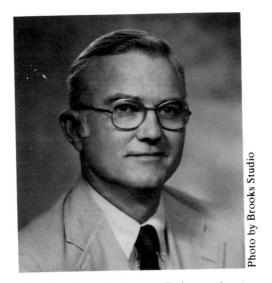

Photo by Brooks Studio

John C. Fletcher, Ph.D., an Episcopal priest, is Assistant for Bioethics in the Warren G. Magnuson Clinical Center of the National Institutes of Health, Bethesda, Maryland. In addition to extensive experience as a counselor, Dr. Fletcher has written widely for medical and professional journals, with special emphasis on moral problems in clinical research, genetic counseling, and prenatal diagnosis.

Dr. Fletcher was president of Inter/Met Seminary in Washington, D.C., and he has been associate professor of church and society at Virginia Theological Seminary in Alexandria.

Coping with Genetic Disorders

Coping with Genetic Disorders

A GUIDE FOR CLERGY AND PARENTS

John C. Fletcher

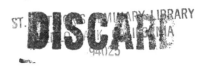

1817

Harper & Row, Publishers, San Francisco
Cambridge, Hagerstown, New York, Philadelphia
London, Mexico City, São Paulo, Sydney

RB
155
F58
1982

This book was written by John C. Fletcher in his private capacity. No official support or endorsement by the National Institutes of Health or of the Department of Health and Human Services is intended or should be inferred.

The case histories and examples in this book are based on actual situations, but in some instances the cases described are composites of several actual cases and in all instances the names and details about each person have been changed. Thus, situations that clergy and parents might encounter are fairly represented but are not actual.

FIRST EDITION

Designer: Jim Mennick

Library of Congress Cataloging in Publication Data

Fletcher, John C.
COPING WITH GENETIC DISORDERS
    Includes bibliographical references and index.
    1. Genetic counseling. I. Title.
RB155.F58 1982   241'.6425   81-48207
ISBN 0-06-062665-8   AACR2

82 83 84 85 86 10 9 8 7 6 5 4 3 2 1

*To Maxwell Boverman, M.D., a psychiatrist
with whom I have collaborated professionally for years,
most recently as a consultant in bioethical dilemmas.
His example teaches me much about the standards of
faithful companionship and responsibility.*

Contents

Introduction

In my professional career, I have been a parish pastor, a seminary teacher and administrator, and an applied bioethicist. I am lucky that my colleagues are willing to put up with my various interests. As a youth, I was intrigued with medicine, but events and the strong influence of some teachers and pastors led me to an Episcopal seminary. Since that day in 1953, my working life has been a rich kaleidoscope of experiences in congregations, theological education, and, of late, organizing a program in applied bioethics for the Warren G. Magnuson Clinical Center of the National Institutes of Health (NIH). The Clinical Center is a five-hundred-bed research hospital where patients and normal volunteers participate in medical research. I introduce myself in public and in meetings at the NIH as a "minister by background with an interest in bioethics." My overriding professional interest has been to join with others to improve the conditions in which theological students and clergy learn, work, and collaborate with other professionals to help troubled people in human life's many struggles.

I wrote this book to help clergy and parents deal with some issues in bioethics that now arise more frequently in pastoral counseling than they did in the past. These matters come up as parents and prospective parents think about using the newly available knowledge of human genetics to plan their families. Applied human genetics is the technical name for a set of activities that draws upon a steadily growing fund of knowledge about causes, diagnoses, and potential treatment of genetic disorders. This area of medicine has profound implications for the moral and spiritual leadership of pastors.

Applied human genetics encompasses genetic screening programs, genetic counseling, prenatal diagnosis, and treatment of genetic disorders. The content of this book falls mainly into the second and third activities, with a good look at the fourth. The basic components of human genes are being charted by scientists, although far more remains to be understood about genes than has been discovered. Scientists conduct laboratory experiments in which new forms of life are the result of recombining genes from one species with those of another in animals, plants, insects, and bacteria. The media report regularly on advances in "genetic engineering," but not enough attention is paid, in my view, to the many implications for parents and families that applied human genetics has already raised. Obviously, applied human genetics influences the basic concept of parenthood. The practices of applied human genetics should be known by religious leaders who teach about the responsibilities of marriage and parenthood, one of the most traditional functions of religious communities.

Bioethics is a term that has gradually replaced its predecessor, medical ethics, because *bio* (from the Greek word for life, *bios)* signifies that ethical issues arise in all of the life sciences, not only medicine. Bioethics is formally defined as *the systematic search for ethical guidance in the proper use of knowledge gained by science and medicine, especially as that knowledge gained is applied to human beings and their problems.* As an applied bioethicist in a research hospital, I work "in the trenches" with physicians, nurses, patients and their families, and other allied professions in the struggle both to do good medical research and keep good faith with values and principles like truth-telling, justice, and human respect.

I greatly benefit from scholars in ethics who labor in the systematic search for the true meaning of these great values and principles. They work in universities, medical schools, and research institutes, such as the Hastings Center and the Kennedy Institute for Ethics at Georgetown University. They share their insights in writings, conferences, and the formal and informal debates that clarify the issues. In many ways, these scholars are to applied ethics as theological scholars in seminaries are to the practice of ministry.

Although physicians criticize the lack of practical solutions in theoretical ethics, and clergy complain about the lack of realism in seminary studies, the indispensable contribution of scholarship is to the meaning and relevance of the *principles* that ought to guide practices in medicine, research, and ministry. Theories of ethics do not necessarily lead to better solutions of problems, but they do deepen the knowledge and the chosen perspective of those of us whose task it is to try to resolve dilemmas. Unprincipled problem-solvers are usually to be avoided like the plague.

This book attempts to link theory and practice. I want to communicate to clergy especially how important their work is to the health of those who consult them in moral dilemmas and in the great life changes of marriage, birth, and death. I also want to stress certain principles that, in my view, ought to guide these consultations and thereby save them from a shallowness and confusion that, at times, can contribute unwittingly to disaster. The original meaning of the English word "health" is wholeness or soundness of mind, body, and spirit. The word for health derives from the verb "to heal," which in Old High German is the root of the words for wholeness and salvation. The Latin word for health derives from *salus*, also the root of the Latin word for salvation. The interdependence of medicine and ministry is clearly demonstrated in these meanings. Human health, in the encompassing meaning of the term, can be greatly enhanced by increasing the number of clergy and physicians who can communicate about principles and practice.

This book has three purposes. First, it explains to clergy and parents the significance of applied human genetics—genetic screening, genetic counseling, prenatal diagnosis, and genetic therapies. Chapter 1 describes the "state of the art" of these four activities in terms easily understood. The chapter answers the question, "Where are we now and where are we going?" with these matters in lay language. I use several brief case histories to describe how the need for ministry arises in these activities and the dilemmas that they spawn. Chapters 3 and 4 discuss in detail two of the most important opportunities for clergy: premarital counseling, and counseling with a family following the birth of an infant with a serous genetic disorder. Chapter 5 discusses the dynamics of counseling in the moral dilemmas of applied human genetics and gives my own views on the cases in Chapter 1. Chapter 6 describes counseling in decisions that parents must make following prenatal diagnosis. The point of Chapters 3 to 6 is to describe a process of counseling in moral dilemmas that respects the many dimensions of a moral problem and employs the uniqueness of the pastoral relationship as a resource. If the first purpose is successful, the reader will be both more informed about the "what is happening?" question and the "how can I help?" question.

The second purpose of the book is to discuss a concept or model of the pastoral ministry as companionship with others and self and God in the many struggles of human life. In my work as a pastor and with other clergy and seminarians, I notice how confused we become about our work and its meaning. To the extent that the confusion is conceptual, the discussion of companionship in Chapter 2 may prove helpful. The theological foundations for the concept of ministry as faithful companionship are also evident in the final three chapters.

The third purpose of the book is to help clergy and laity with the question of theodicy as it arises in genetic disease. I have had trouble facing this question many times. The question is, "How can God be both good and powerful and yet allow such terrible diseases to happen to innocent children?" Chapters 7 to 9 speak to this question. Clergy, more than others, have the "why?" question put to them in the midst of terrible suffering. My way of thinking about God's power and goodness, as well as about biological evolution, tries to hold together all that is known by the scientific study of genetic disease and all that I can believe about God with intellectual honesty and moral integrity. Chapter 9 closes with a discussion of the possibility of genetic therapies and encouragement of this goal.

Because this book has a practical purpose, I do not reference each idea or association that I gleaned from the academics. I simply state here how much I owe intellectually to a great teacher of ethics, H. Richard Niebuhr, with whom I never had the opportunity to study, and to his charismatic brother, Reinhold Niebuhr, whose friendship and encouragement I prized in the last years of his life. I owe the Virginia Theological Seminary a debt of gratitude for supporting my graduate studies (1964–1966) in Christian ethics. I find Daniel Day Williams, Schubert Ogden, John B. Cobb, Jr., and other theologians influenced by process thought to be creative links between theology, ethics, and biology. I am sure that this is true because of their appreciation of the role of biological and cultural evolution in human life and thought.

James Gustafson, Stephen Toulmin, and Daniel Callahan have each influenced my thinking about bioethics, especially by their criticism of ethical absolutism and by their mediating approach to the issues. Joseph Fletcher (who is a friend, but not a relative) helps me remember always to weigh the facts that can be known in each dilemma before finally invoking the ethical ought.

Many physicians instructed me on medical genetics in research groups at the Hastings Center, and in clinics, conferences, and rounds in various hospitals. I must thank especially W. French Anderson and Robert Murray. I have learned from both of these generous and thoughtful men for more than ten years. Joseph Schulman, Duane Alexander, and Mark Evans of the National Institute of Child Health and Human Development give me many hours to clarify the social policy implications of human genetic studies. I profit from Aubrey Milunsky's writings, both scientific and popular. He generously provided most of the figures that appear in Chapter 1, and I draw upon his clear explanations in many places. Sandra Schlesinger, genetic counselor at the Clinical Center, advised with the content of Chapter 1, provided an interesting case for Chapter 3, and helped to reconstruct the Family Health History Chart.

My supervisor, Mortimer B. Lipsett, Director of the Clinical Center, and the former and current Deputy Directors, Griff T. Ross and Jay Shapiro, encourage and support my work in applied bioethics. I am fortunate to have the services of a psychiatric consultant who is in private practice, Maxwell Boverman, in launching a new program in bioethics. He helps me understand the interpersonal aspects of ethical conflicts and guides me in the role conflicts that are part of any interdisciplinary work. His independent spirit and honesty have been invaluable to me and the institution.

In the field of pastoral studies, I am indebted to James Adams, Rector of St. Mark's Episcopal Church in Washington, D. C., a congregation to which I and my family gladly belong. Loren Mead, Director of the Alban Institute, urged me to write this book and made many helpful comments on earlier drafts, as did Celia Hahn, a caring editor of work intended for clergy. David Baker, once an intern at the Clinical Center and now a Presbyterian minister, helped me with the initial outline and objectives of the book. My former colleagues in Inter/Met Seminary (1970–1977) created the ideal setting to learn about the practice of ministry in congregations in a metropolitan area. The best hope for the pastoral ideals of that experiment in theological education is that they live on in the persons of the graduates and friends in seminaries and foundations who contributed to the work of those intense years.

John Shopp of Harper & Row read an earlier version of the manuscript and advised changes that greatly improved it. My thanks go to Cheryl Hailey who typed the final manuscript and to Pat Loy who typed preliminary drafts. Nelson Chipchin, a volunteer at the Clinical Center, read every word of the draft and helped me simplify the contents.

My wife, Dale, has helped me in so many ways for so many years by her steadiness and hard work. The dilemmas in this book were subjects of *ad hoc* seminars with her and our children, Caldwell, Page, and Adele. I am especially grateful to our family for the close companionship that is indispensable for one who aspires to be a faithful companion to others in science, ethics, and ministry.

I

A GUIDE FOR CLERGY AND PARENTS TO APPLIED HUMAN GENETICS

I. What Is Applied Human Genetics?

Why should clergy and parents be interested in human genetics? Anything new and reputedly so complex must take time and energy. Why not let someone else worry about it? Geneticist Aubrey Milunsky points out that the most important reason for knowing about genes is that each person carries between four and eight faulty genes.[1] We may either already have a genetic disorder, develop one at a later time, or transmit a disorder to one or more of our children. Each person's self-interest demands being informed. We also need to know what can be done to discover if we are carriers of a specific disorder, and, if so, if a disorder can be diagnosed in the developing fetus early enough to enable us to choose a course of action.

Another reason why clergy and parents need to know is so that we can do our best in the existing choices about what *ought* to be done to identify carriers and diagnose genetic disorders. Because something *can* be done is not a good reason why it *ought* to be done. A diagnosis does not automatically determine what ought to be done. As human beings, we decide these matters by drawing on our ethical beliefs, feelings, and education. Most people feel better after making difficult choices if they are able to say, "I did everything I could reasonably do," especially if the choice is between two bad options. Clergy are obligated to be reliable guides in moral dilemmas. Parents are obligated to protect their children and their families from harm and to give them the greatest chance to develop their potential. Both clergy and parents need to be informed about genetics in order to fulfill their obligations.*

In the United States, at least one in ten individuals, or over 20 million people, now have or will develop an inherited disorder. Over three thousand genetic disorders have been identified to date, and the list grows. These disorders account for 25 to 30 percent of admissions to children's hospitals. About three to four of every hundred infants born have some major birth defect, and over six million people in the United States are mentally retarded due to hereditary reasons. As the reader works through the information that follows, these questions may help to sift it for what is especially relevant:

- What do I need to know to protect myself and my family from harm?
- What do I need to know to counsel others wisely and refer them to genetic counseling?
- What should I know to participate intelligently in debates about the social and ethical questions raised by applied human genetics?

What Are Genes?

To answer this question, the reader must be able to distinguish between cells, genes, and chromosomes. A human body is a living network of billions of *cells*. We continue living because, as millions of cells die each second, they are replaced. Some cells die faster than others and are rapidly replaced. Brain cells are nonreplaceable, but die slowly. Most cells have their own special function. For example, cells in the liver produce what the liver needs to function, and brain cells make what memory requires biochemically. Each cell has a nucleus, a center of operations, or a kind of headquarters. The nucleus contains tiny threads called *chromosomes*, made up of chemical compounds. These chromosomes are themselves composed of *genes*, which are the building blocks of chromosomes and

---

* A glossary of terms to help the reader is provided in Appendix A. Rather than explaining each disease when it is mentioned in the text, brief definitions are given in Appendix A, along with other terms in human genetics.

thus of heredity. The chromosomes, with their component genes, are blueprints for the future of human organisms that are passed on in sexual reproduction. We receive one-half of our genes from each of our parents. Each gene has a "program" that has been shaped through evolution and has its own part to play in making us what we are. The environment in which we grow, with its culture and special characteristics, interacts with the genes to comprise the larger framework of human growth and development.

I found a jewel of an analogy in a book by Richard Dawkins,[2] a British zoologist, that helped me understand the transmission of genes from parent to child. Dawkins likens the human body with its thousand million cells to a gigantic library containing many rooms. Every cell comprises one room in the building. In each room (that is, cell) there is a bookcase (that is, nucleus) that contains the architect's plans for the entire building. Dawkins says, "Incidentally, of course there is no architect. The plans have been assembled by natural selection."[3] (The concept of natural selection will be discussed in Chapter 9.) The plans are printed in forty-six volumes (that is, chromosomes). Chromosomes can be seen microscopically as long threads with the invisible genes strung out upon them. The genes are analogous to "pages" in the volumes. Genes are composed of DNA molecules, and these can be likened to printed words on the page, or the messages themselves. DNA molecules are chains of nucleic acids too small to be seen by a microscope, but elegantly imagined by James D. Watson and Francis Crick,[4] with the help of X-ray diffraction photography, as a "double helix," a pair of nucleotide chains coiled together in a spiral. If one imagines the helix as a spiral staircase, then the steps of the stairs are composed of two paired molecules (see Figure 1).

To return to the library image, the letters that compose the words on each page, or the alphabet used by the architect, begin with the combinations of four nucleic acids that always pair with their opposites. These four building block letters are *adenine, thymine, cytosine* and *guanine,* simply shortened to A, T, C, and G. These four nucleotides comprise two groups of molecules, the purines (A and G) and the pyramidines (T and C). If the instructions for making these building blocks, the genes, are correct, they will be correct in every room of the library. If the instructions for any gene are incorrect in

Fig. 1. Schematic diagram of the DNA double helix

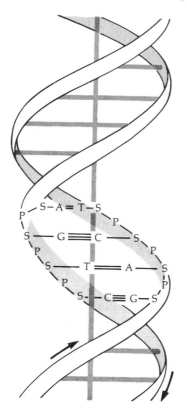

The backbone of each helical chain is made up of alternating deoxyribose sugar (S) and phosphate (P). The two chains are joined by weak interactions between the nucleotide bases adenine (A), thymine (T), cytosine (C), and guanine (G). Adenine-thymine pairs are held together by two hydrogen bonds, while cytosine-guanine pairs are joined by three such bonds.

SOURCE: Walter F. Bodmer and Luisi L. Cavalli-Sforza, *Genetics, Evolution and Man* (San Francisco: W. H. Freeman and Company). Copyright © 1976.

one room, they will be incorrect in every room. The basic reasons why genetic disorders occur is that, for any of a number of causes, incorrect instructions are given at the building block level.

How Are Genes Transmitted from Parents to Child?

For centuries, people wondered why children of the same parents looked so much alike yet were different in important features. This variability in humans, as well as in every other species, was not understood until the true number and size of the chromosomes (from the Greek words for "color" and "body") were known. The chromosomes within a cell's nucleus, as seen through a microscope, look essentially like the shapes in Figure 2, enlarged thousands of times. The chromosomes pictured in a photograph can be cut out by order of size from largest to smallest. If they are normal, they look like those in Figure 3.

Fig. 2. Chromosomes within a cell as seen through the microscope

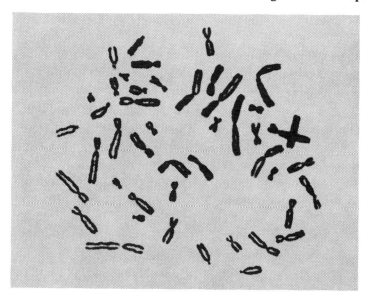

SOURCE: Aubrey Milunsky, *Know Your Genes* (Boston: Houghton Mifflin, 1977). Copyright © 1977 by Aubrey Milunsky, M.D. Reprinted by permission of Houghton Mifflin Company.

In Figure 3, we can count twenty-two pairs of chromosomes and one pair of X (or sex) chromosomes, meaning the sex is female. If the sex were male, there would be one X and one Y at the twenty-third chromosome. Since the Y is very short, as compared to the X, geneticists arrange it at the end of the size sequence, as shown in Figure 4.

Fig. 3. Normal human chromosomes in one cell, arranged in descending order of size

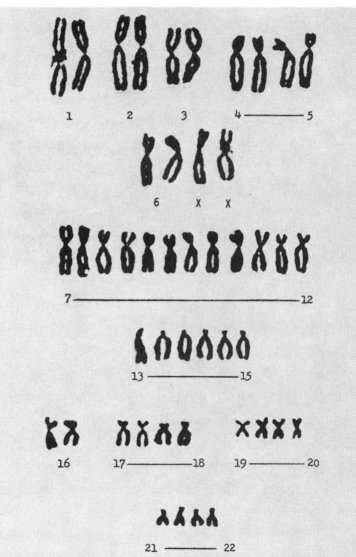

SOURCE: Aubrey Milunsky, *Know Your Genes* (Boston: Houghton Mifflin, 1977).

Fig. 4. Normal human chromosomes from one cell arranged in descending order of size

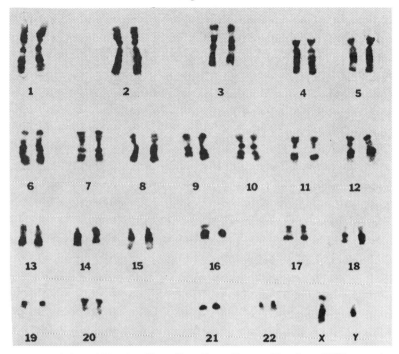

SOURCE: Aubrey Milunsky, *Know Your Genes* (Boston: Houghton Mifflin, 1977).

Every cell in the human body, except the sex cells, has forty-six chromosomes. Sperm and eggs, which are made in the testes and ovaries, have twenty-three cells, which is fortunate since reproduction could otherwise not occur. The process by which sex cells are made is called *meiosis*, derived from the Greek word for reduction. Figure 5 shows the six steps of the process by which gametes (sperm and eggs) are the result.

The genetic composition of each sperm and egg is different. The uniqueness of each human being has often been illustrated by the example of fingerprints, but fingerprints are just a gross example of the uniqueness of the individual. Each sperm and egg is a unique event. Each parent is capable of producing more than 19 trillion

Fig. 5. Chromosome division (meiosis) step by step

Step 1: one cell with a pair of chromosomes.
Step 2: the chromosomes split lengthwise and begin to pair off.
Step 3: the cell nucleus begins to divide.
Step 4: the cell nucleus and the cell that it occupies have divided into two new nuclei, each containing a pair of chromosomes.
Step 5: the two chromosomes in each new nucleus now begin to move apart as the cell and its nucleus divide.
Step 6: a new cell and nucleus are formed, each with only one chromosome from the preceding cell. These are the sperm cells or the egg. Each has twenty-three chromosomes.

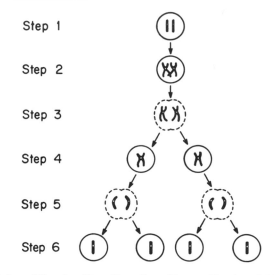

SOURCE: Aubrey Milunsky, *Know Your Genes* (Boston: Houghton Mifflin, 1977).

different combinations of genes, so it is very unlikely that even one of these combinations would exactly copy the genetic makeup of any ancestor.

The library analogy helps us to understand how sex cells are one of a kind genetically, as well as being the source of many accidents in the events of meiosis that lead to genetic disorders. The uniqueness comes about because, during the making of a sperm or egg, pieces of each chromosome from the father change places with the exactly matching pieces of chromosomes from the mother. Recall Dawkins's idea that the forty-six chromosomes are like forty-six volumes in the bookcases (nuclei) of each cell. The idea is a bit more complicated than simply single volumes. To be exact, the forty-six volumes consist of twenty-three *matched volumes*. The pages of the volumes can be imagined as loose-leaf binders. During meiosis, pages from one volume are swapped with those from the matching volume. The result is a complete "sex cell library" composed of equal bits of forty-six volumes, but now comprising twenty-three volumes. To make another complete library, that sex cell library must await the time of reproduction. At fertilization, the new individual receives one cell with twenty-three chromosomes from each parent, which constitute one new cell with forty-six chromosomes. The developing human body stores these cells for the future. This scrambling process in meiosis is called recombination or "crossing-over." Crossing-over is the greatest cause of the vast variety in nature. Recombination does not make new genes; rather, it makes never before seen combinations of old genes. Each person's genes were prepared in the testes and ovaries of parents and grandparents.

What Causes Genetic Disorders?

Many things can go wrong in the making and transmission of chromosomes from parents to child. These are called *chromosomal abnormalities*. Chromosomes in the sperm or egg can be abnormal at fertilization. Sometimes chromosomes stick together, making a disorder. The chromosomes may have a defective structure or break abnormally. Part of a chromosome may be deleted. Probably between 45 and 50 percent of all conceptions are spontaneously aborted because of chromosomal abnormalities. The human body, via the chromosomes, it would appear, has a sensitive way of screening the new embryo for serious problems.

A second source of trouble is an *abnormal process of cell division* that results in too many or too few chromosomes. Figure 6 shows

Fig. 6. Cell division (mitosis)

Step 1: a single cell with a pair of chromosomes.
Step 2: the chromosomes split lengthwise and make a total of two pairs.
Step 3: the chromosome pairs separate; the cell nucleus and
         the cell itself begin to divide.
Step 4: one chromosome member of each pair is found in a new cell.

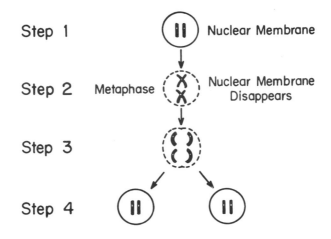

SOURCE: Aubrey Milunsky, *Know Your Genes* (Boston: Houghton Mifflin, 1977).

the normal process of *mitosis* or cell division that must occur in every cell.

An illustration of abnormal cell division is shown in Figure 7, in this case in the ovary, although the same problem can occur in sperm. Figure 7 contains every step of Figure 6 down to Step 5. At this point, the cell nucleus and the cell that it occupies begin to divide into two, but here the chromosome pair fails to separate. Both chromosomes remain in one cell, in this case, in the egg. The other cell, represented in Figure 7 at Step 6 by the empty circle, has all of the other chromosomes except the missing one. Most commonly, this is chromosome number 21. So some cells have an extra chromosome 21 and some have none. Scientists think that the cell division problem may occur at Step 3 or 4. At any rate, when the sperm and egg fertilize, the result is that many cells in the new embryo will have an extra chromosome 21. The result is a disorder known as Down syndrome, which can involve serious retardation and other physical problems.

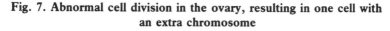

Fig. 7. Abnormal cell division in the ovary, resulting in one cell with an extra chromosome

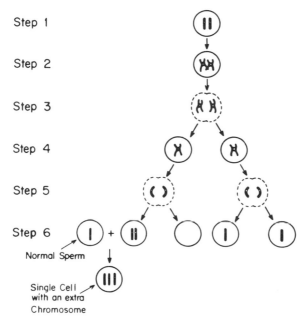

SOURCE: Aubrey Milunsky, *Know Your Genes* (Boston: Houghton Mifflin, 1977).

A third cause of genetic disorders is a so-called *inborn error of metabolism*. The wrong message is sent by one or more genes, making a biochemical defect that results in a deficiency or accumulation of substances. Sometimes these disorders are carried more frequently in specific ethnic groups or are related to circumscribed geographical locations. One in every twenty-five Caucasians in the United States is a carrier of a recessive gene for cystic fibrosis. One in each ten black Americans is a carrier of a recessive gene for sickle cell disease. If these carriers reproduce with other carriers of the same recessive gene, there is a 25 percent risk in each pregnancy of producing an affected child.

A fourth source of genetic disorders is *mutations*. These events are spontaneous changes in the genes, in which the harmful gene is not inherited but occurs *de novo*—anew in the affected individual. Most mutations happen either randomly or for reasons that are not understood. Mutations are also caused by irradiation from X-rays, atomic energy, and the atmosphere. Once the gene is changed permanently by a mutation, all of the benefit or harm that results is copied in every other cell of the individual in whom the change has taken place, and is also inherited by the offspring.

The four causes of genetic disorders presented thus far are clearly genetic. There is a fifth cause, *multifactorial*, meaning a combination of genetic and environmental causes. Case 4, presented later in this chapter, illustrates this type.

What Are the Risks of Inheriting or Transmitting a Genetic Disorder?

A person who wants to answer this question must first know the family health history of the parents. Based on this information, a primary physician can make a referral concerning genetic counseling. Genetic counseling is a service provided in most large cities, certainly in all states, by qualified physicians or other health professionals. If difficulty is encountered obtaining a referral from a physician, it is advisable to telephone the local chapter of the March of Dimes Birth Defects Foundation, a national organization that readily provides information and access to genetic counseling. If there is a possibility of risk of inheritance or transmission, a genetic counselor should be consulted without delay.

Persons may need genetic counseling if they:

- are concerned about their family health history and need information
- have a genetic condition that may affect their reproduction or the health of a child (e.g., being a carrier for one or more genetic disorders)
- have a known risk related to reproduction

- want to understand their options in case of genetic risks (e.g., adoption, prenatal diagnosis, elective abortion, artificial insemination, etc.)
- want help to educate other members of the family as to genetic risks and the consequences of disease

There are several modes of inheritance of genetic disorders. Geneticists refer to them as *dominant, recessive, sex-linked,* and *multifactorial.* Having mentioned another mode, mutation, let us briefly review those, with the help of case reports. The first three cases are true, but the facts and names have been disguised. Case 4 is based upon events occurring with more frequency in the United States. I discuss my own view of these cases in Chapter 5.

Dominant Inheritance

Case 1. Who Is Too Young for Genetic Counseling?

The clergyperson in a congregation was consulted by Jane, who had been divorced from Ted for three years. They have two daughters, ages fourteen and twelve. Ted's father had Huntington's disease, signs of which began to appear in his late thirties. This disease involves neurological changes that affect the body, and usually results in severe loss of mental capacities and death. Ted has a 50 percent chance of inheriting the disease, which is carried by a dominant gene, but to date he has no symptoms. Jane, who has legal custody of the girls, wanted advice from the pastor about whether she should take them to physicians to learn about their risk of also having Huntington's disease. She asked the pastor, "Do you think it is right to expose them to these facts? Will it frighten them too much? Why should they know about a disease they might have for which there is no known cure? They are young, but the oldest is old enough to date."

Figure 8 depicts the way a dominant disorder is inherited. One affected parent, in this case the father, has a faulty gene inherited from his father that dominates its normal counterpart contributed by his mother. Each of his children has a 50 percent chance of inheriting either the defective gene (D) or the normal gene (n). There are hundreds of dominant disorders. They can come from either father or mother. Clergy probably will be aware of families in which deafness, blindness, and short stature appear. These conditions are often caused by a dominant disorder.

Recessive Inheritance

Case 2. Should a Therapeutic Lie Be Condoned?

A minister was asked for counseling by a woman in his congregation. She and her husband had two children. The first child was normal. The second suffered from a disease that can be transmitted only when both parents are carriers of a recessive gene. Following the discovery that the child had the disease, the physician asked both parents to have a blood test for the carrier state. The woman's test revealed that she was positive (i.e., a carrier). However, her husband's test was negative. Before notifying the father, the physician asked her, in private, if she could clarify the situation. She admitted to him that she had had intercourse with another man several times in the same month the affected child was conceived. Her husband did not know of her extramarital affair, and he assumed the child was his own. The physician had not yet formulated an answer to the couple about their carrier tests, and he asked the woman if she desired him to tell the truth or to tell a "therapeutic lie." The lie would consist of explaining the father's negative result by saying that there was a "fresh mutation" in him that contributed to the disease. The physician said that he would leave the matter in her hands to decide. She asked the minister for help, afraid that her husband might harm her or the child if the truth were known, but also afraid that she was contributing to his false belief that he was a carrier, a state of affairs that could harm him emotionally and even financially, if an employer were to misunderstand the meaning of carrier status. What ought the minister do with this information?

Figure 9 shows how recessive inheritance happens. Both parents carry a gene that, in them, generally causes little or no harm. When they have a child, there is a 25 percent chance in each pregnancy that the child will have the disease. There is a 50 percent chance that the child will be a carrier of one recessive gene. The normal gene in the carrier (N) overrides the damage that can be done by the

Fig. 8. Dominant inheritance

(a)

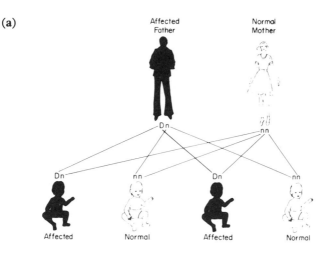

Affected Father   Normal Mother

Dn   nn

Dn   nn   Dn   nn

Affected   Normal   Affected   Normal

(a). One affected parent (of either sex) has a defective gene (D) that dominates its normal counterpart (n). Every child has a 50 percent chance of inheriting either the defective gene D (and will then have the disease) or the normal gene n from the affected parent.

(b). A typical family tree of dominant inheritance, and seen, for example, in Huntington's disease, heart disease due to hyper-cholesterolemia, and hundreds of other disorders.

(b)

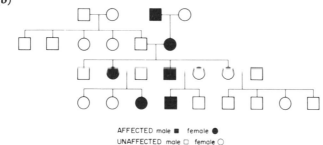

AFFECTED male ■ female ●
UNAFFECTED male □ female ○

SOURCE: Aubrey Milunsky, *Know Your Genes* (Boston: Houghton Mifflin, 1977).

problem gene (r), but when two recessive genes (r) coincide in the infant, the disease results. Cystic fibrosis, sickle cell disease, and Tay-Sachs disease are common recessive disorders (see the Glossary of Terms for descriptions of these diseases).

Sex-Linked Disorders

Case 3. Consequences of a Sex-Linked Disorder

A pastoral counselor of a Protestant denomination was called for an appointment by a woman in her fifth month of pregnancy, who identified herself as a "Catholic with a serious problem." Because the woman felt she could not go to her priest, the counselor agreed to see her. She came to the office crying and appeared despondent. She said that she had a son with Lesch-Nyhan disease, a genetic disorder transmitted to males by their mothers. She had not known that she was a carrier, since she was the only child in her family. The disease causes involuntary biting and self-mutilation of the fingers and lips, mental retardation, and usually leads to death before twenty. She felt "terrible" about this baby, and she and her husband abstained from intercourse until she learned that a new technique called amniocentesis* could be used during pregnancy to diagnose the disease. She lived in a strongly Catholic community and had heard her priest criticize amniocentesis as abortion-related. Nevertheless, she and her husband had traveled to another city and had amniocentesis with a second pregnancy. A healthy girl was born. She confided in the priest later, during confession, that she had taken this step. He remarked that she had entered into temptation but had been saved from having to decide literally about abortion. He kept her confidence and her daughter was baptized. She explained that she became pregnant again, "because my husband wants a normal boy so badly and so do I." She traveled to a city for genetic diagnosis. She had just heard from the clinic that the news was bad. A male fetus with the disease had been

---

*A medical procedure, performed between the sixteenth and eighteenth week of pregnancy, by which a needle is inserted into the uterus and a sample of amniotic fluid is withdrawn. Analysis of fetal cells in the amniotic fluid can indicate problems in the unborn child.

Fig. 9. Recessive inheritance

(a)

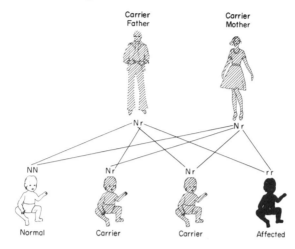

(a). Both parents are usually healthy, but each carries a defective gene that by itself generally causes no problems. Disease follows when a person receives 2 of these recessive genes. There is a 25 percent chance that a person will inherit a double dose of the defective gene; a 50 percent chance of being a carrier; and a 25 percent chance of being neither a carrier nor affected.

(b). A typical family tree of recessive inheritance, and seen in cystic fibrosis. Note that there were no previously affected individuals in the family. However, if one looks into the distant past of the families involved, cousin marriages are not unusual.

(b)

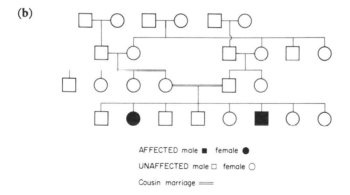

AFFECTED male ■ female ●

UNAFFECTED male □ female ○

Cousin marriage ══

SOURCE: Aubrey Milunsky, *Know Your Genes* (Boston: Houghton Mifflin, 1977).

diagnosed. She said to the counselor, "My husband and I have decided to have an abortion. My problem is that I probably should also have my tubes tied at the same time, so this awful thing won't happen again. But then I will never have the son we want so much. What should I do?"

Figure 10 describes how the sex- or X-linked mode of inheritance occurs. The problem gene is carried on one of the X chromosomes of the mother, who inherited it from her mother. Because she has one normal gene at the location on the other X chromosome inherited from her father, she is healthy. But when she and her husband conceive and the X chromosome with the problem is transmitted to a boy, there is no other X chromosome to cancel out the damage. The risk for the boys of having the disease is 50 percent. For the girls, there will be a 50 percent risk of being a carrier. The best-known disorders that are transmitted this way are hemophilia, muscular dystrophy, and Lesch-Nyhan disease. If the affected male reproduces, there is a 100 percent chance that all of the daughters will be carriers, assuming that the mother is normal. Both men and women are involved in the transmission of X-linked disease.

Multiple Factors

Case 4. Who Is the Pastor to Help?

A pastor in a rural, mountainous area of the Southeast made the church education rooms available to a traveling genetics clinic sponsored by the state university medical school. The state paid a monthly rental fee that was not high but helped the small church meet its financial problems. A team of physicians, nurses, and a genetic associate visited at intervals of four months to see patients and families referred by other physicians for genetic disorders. The pastor came to know the physician better as the months passed, and the physician asked the pastor one day if he would be willing to stay after the clinic to meet with her and the parents of a two-year-old child with *spina bifida* who had recently died in the university hospital. The physician explained that this disorder is now the leading cause of paralysis in children. She showed the pastor a picture of a newborn with an open neural tube defect and explained that, with

Fig. 10. Sex-linked (X-linked) inheritance

(a)

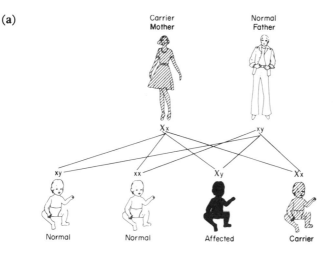

(a). The defective gene is carried on one X chromosome of the mother, who is usually healthy. Disease follows when that X chromosome containing the defective gene is transmitted to a male. The odds for each male child is 50/50 for being affected, while 50 percent of the daughters will be carriers.

(b). A typical family tree of X-linked disease such as hemophilia or muscular dystrophy.

(b)

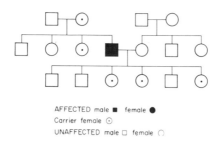

AFFECTED male ■   female ●
Carrier female ⊙
UNAFFECTED male □   female ○

SOURCE: Aubrey Milunsky, *Know Your Genes* (Boston: Houghton Mifflin, 1977).

this condition, the spinal column does not develop correctly. Although open lesions can be closed with surgery, most children will have serious problems all their lives and perhaps die, as did the child of this couple (see Figure 11). New techniques of blood tests for pregnant women now exist, explained the physician, that can detect the possibility of spina bifida in pregnancy, but other tests with more sophisticated methods must follow to confirm it. The problem for the couple, the wife again pregnant, is that two blood tests have been positive and therefore suspicious. She advised the couple to travel to the university center for more tests with ultrasound, and possibly amniocentesis. The couple refused, saying that they "didn't want any more to do with doctors. The Lord gives and the Lord takes away." The physician added that she believes the problem is that they are terribly frightened and still grieving for their lost child, and blame her. They are also at a higher risk of having another child with spina bifida. She knows that the couple are not members of his church, but will the pastor help her by meeting with the parents to discuss the implications of their refusal?

This case illustrates problems associated with a type of disorder that has multifactorial causes. Ancestry, climate, geography, nutrition, and seasonal effects are probably factors in the inheritance of spina bifida.

Other birth defects that fall into this multifactorial category include cleft palate, club feet, pyloric stenosis (a congenital block where the stomach extends into the intestine), certain heart defects, and dislocated hips.[5] For all of the problems mentioned here, if either of the parents are affected or if one child has been previously born with such a problem, there is a much higher risk of having a subsequently affected child.

Can Genetic Disorders Be Prevented or Treated?

For centuries, the main form of prevention of genetic disorder was negative social action. Only restraint from procreation and prohibition by marriage laws or customs prevented genetic disorders. Our ancestors were more the victims of fate and necessity than we are, since today there are scientifically reliable ways to get infor-

Fig. 11. Spina bifida

Normal spine is shown on the left. On the right, the neural tube has failed to close and the spinal cord and nerve bundles protrude through the baby's back. (Drawing by Jane Walsh.)

Normal spine   Myelomeningocele

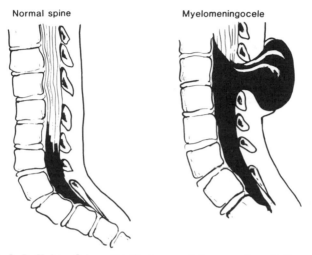

SOURCE: G. B. Kolata, *Science* 209 (Sept. 12, 1980), pp. 1216–1218. Copyright © 1980 by the American Association for the Advancement of Science.

mation about oneself, family members, and also the developing fetus that create new alternatives for action.

Genetic Screening

Physicians do genetic screening for three reasons. First, screening can uncover a disorder that is actual or latent, and treatment or support can be offered. Second, screening can detect people of reproductive age who are at risk to transmit a genetic disorder, and information can be given to these persons for planning reproduction. Third, scientists need to answer questions about the natural history of a disorder, how frequently it appears in the population, and how the gene(s) for the disorder is distributed.

The most prevalent use of genetic screening follows birth, when the blood or urine of the new baby can be tested. Biochemical disorders such as PKU (phenylketonuria) can be diagnosed in a few hours and therapy (diet, in this case) begun that prevents serious retardation. PKU is caused by the incorrect message of one or more genes that omit the production of an enzyme. As a result, if the newborn is fed milk that has a high content of phenylalanine, and the missing enzyme cannot do its work of breaking down this substance, the child's brain will be affected and retardation will follow. A substitute diet of synthetic milk products is used. PKU happens in about one in fifteen thousand births.

As the list of conditions (most of them more rare than PKU) for which newborns can be screened has grown, so has controversy about whether the effort is worth it. New York's legislature passed a law in 1974 requiring that all new babies be screened for seven disorders: PKU, maple sugar urine disease, homocystinuria, histidinemia, galactosemia, adenosine deaminase deficiency (ADD), and sickle cell anemia. Objections have been raised to screening for three of these.[6] Some scientists wonder if histidinemia (elevated histidine in blood) is really a disease. Found in only one in twenty-five thousand births, and at times associated with mental retardation, it is treatable by diet, but there is no evidence that a diet changes the condition. There is no treatment for ADD, a very rare disease, and screening all infants (white or black) for sickle cell disease, when only ten percent are at risk, does not seem to be cost effective.

Other controversial newborn screening includes that for chromosomal disorders for which no treatment exists and for chromosome patterns (XYY) linked to antisocial behavior by disputed evidence. Clergy and parents should know the practices of the state in which they reside prior to birth of infants, so that the informed consent process, required where there are laws, can be meaningful rather than an empty gesture. Parents should also know that false positive results can occasionally happen because of laboratory or human error.

Physicians and public health authorities have organized two large-scale screening programs since the early 1970s for adults and young people old enough to reproduce. One was for Tay-Sachs carrier screening, a recessive trait that leads to brain damage so severe as to be lethal in the first two or three years of life. Tragically, the infants appear to be normal for six months to one year. This disease occurs with a higher frequency (one in 3600 births) among Ashkenazi Jews whose ancestry is in Middle Europe than in the non-Jewish population (one in 360,000 births). Individuals and couples can be screened for the recessive condition by a simple and inexpensive blood test, informed about the results, and if found positive (i.e., carrier) they can be counseled about their options in reproduction. Some Jewish leaders are concerned about "overselling" mass screening for a so-called Jewish disease, citing possible psychological damage to younger carriers who might feel stigmatized. Some Jewish authorities are concerned about the abortion issue, while others are worried about the low response to screening because only 10 to 15 percent of the most affected age group in any U.S. community responded.

It is important to note that not only Ashkenazi Jews suffer from Tay-Sachs disease. In North America, among non-Jews, there are between one and two carriers for each 300 to 400 persons. In Western Newfoundland, Tay-Sachs disease is found among those persons of British descent whose ancestors inhabited the island for more than two hundred years. To the extent that mistaken ideas about disease could exacerbate anti-Semitism, some knowledge of these facts can help.

Likewise, early efforts to mandate screening for the sickle cell trait were very controversial and even counterproductive. Beginning in 1970, many state legislators rushed to frame laws mandating screening for black children. Unfortunately, there was some confusion about the difference between a genetic carrier trait (the carrier will hardly ever manifest signs of the disease) and the disease itself. In part, even medical literature was caught up in the confusion, in that an editorial referred to screening "22 million Afro-Americans" for a "dread disease."[7] People who were screened were bombarded with faulty information and often received their test results by postcard. Some black sickle cell trait carriers were unjustly barred from sports, denied employment, or discharged from jobs. Damage was done despite the best intentions of genetic screeners, summarized in a set of guidelines that probably came too late to prevent the worst harm.[8]

As with Tay-Sachs disease, medical ignorance of sickle cell disease can increase racial or ethnic prejudice. It is important to know that not only blacks are carriers of a recessive gene for sickle cell disease. Peoples whose ancestry descends from regions where malaria was or is still prevalent tend to carry this trait, which at one time may have increased their resistance to malaria. Thus Greeks, Egyptians, Italians and citizens of India, Southeast Asia, and other tropical climates are also affected by the disorder. The gene for the carrier trait, before the mosquito was defeated by pesticide, conferred a biological advantage. This gene became more frequent in later generations, because carriers lived longer and reproduced. Now a casualty of culture, the gene causes more harm than good.

A newer form of screening pregnancies for neural tube defects is now possible. When the neural tube remains open, an enzyme made only by the fetus, alpha-fetoprotein (AFP), leaks into the circulatory system of the mother. Her obstetrician-gynecologist gives a blood test in the fourth month of pregnancy that detects a higher AFP level than normal. If confirmed by a second test, the mother is referred quickly for further studies using ultrasound, a method of visualizing the fetus by way of sound waves transmitted onto a screen. Ultrasound is used to rule out twins, the death of the fetus, or other reasons that may lead to a high AFP level. If these are omitted, physicians may proceed to take fluid from the *amnion*, the sac in which the fetus grows, and sample it for AFP levels. If this final step shows a higher AFP, the chances are very high that a neural tube defect is present. In Great Britain, it has become routine to screen almost every pregnancy for neural tube defects. In the United States, screening is done on a smaller scale in a very few areas. Due to controversy about the ethical, legal, and social implications of screening, the Food and Drug Administration has not yet released rules for drug companies to market the procedure used by laboratories for assaying the mother's blood. It remains to be seen if the rules for physicians, laboratories and drug companies will be strict, flexible, or nonexistent. The major concern is that the woman be counseled wisely about the steps involved, and that the additional services (ultrasound, amniocentesis) be quickly available.

The number of genetic disorders and carrier states for which one can be screened changes from year to year. Who should be most interested in being screened? In Milunsky's view,[9] parents or prospective parents may be advised to consult a physician if one of five reasons appear: (1) one parent has a genetic disorder; (2) The parents have a child with a hereditary disorder; (3) there is a family history of a genetic disorder; (4) the individual is automatically a carrier (e.g., the daughter of a father with hemophilia); or (5) the individual belongs to an ethnic group with higher risks for a specific genetic disease (e.g., blacks of African origin, Jews of Ashkenazic origin, or Greeks from coastal regions).

Prenatal Diagnosis

There are additional reasons to the five listed above as to why parents may seek advice about prenatal diagnosis. There is a higher risk of mental retardation associated with children born to older couples, when the mother is above thirty-seven years of age. To detect Down syndrome, many physicians advise amniocentesis after the mother is thirty-five years of age; but the statistical risk becomes significant at thirty-seven. The mother may have been exposed to X-rays, drugs, or some other agent during pregnancy. She may have had one or more spontaneous abortions in previous pregnancies, suggesting that there were chromosomal disorders. These are the accepted medical reasons for seeking prenatal diagnosis. Two other controversial reasons may occasionally arise. The parents may feel unduly anxious about their chances of having a retarded child and want to rule out one or more disorders. Or they may want to know the sex of the fetus, with no reason beyond planning the birth order of children, or because several children of the same gender may have already been born. The latter request remains unusual to date, but if the clergy serve communities in which there are significant Asian, Middle Eastern, or Indian populations, there may be such requests because of strong male preference. (A list of the disorders that can currently be diagnosed prenatally is provided in Appendix B.)

Since the late 1960s, *amniocentesis* has been the most used technique for prenatal diagnosis of genetic disorders. The term *amniocentesis* comes from *amnio* (amniotic fluid) and *centesis* (puncture). By needle puncture of the amniotic fluid between the sixteenth and eighteenth weeks of pregnancy, fetal cells can be obtained and cultured in the laboratory for diagnostic purposes. Virtually all of the known chromosomal disorders can be diagnosed by amniocentesis. Many sex-linked disorders and metabolic disorders can also be diagnosed. Amniocentesis has become so widely used that some obstetricians now do the procedure in the office as opposed to an outpatient procedure in the hospital. The most significant risk of amniocentesis, fetal death from infection or needle puncture, is about 0.5 percent or 1 in 200 in the United States and Canada today. Errors in prenatal diagnosis occur rarely, but parents should also know that the accuracy rate for diagnosis is not perfect. In about five out of one thousand cases, the results are misdiagnosed due to human error; it can also happen that the fetus has another disorder than the one being studied.

A second method using needle puncture with *fetoscopy* enables a physician to see the fetus or remove a tissue sample for biopsy or blood for testing. In fetoscopy, a small-gauge endoscope is inserted into the abdomen of the pregnant woman. Ultrasound precedes the insertion to ensure correct positioning of the endoscope and to enable the physician to avoid the placenta. With a fetoscope, an abnormal number of fingers and toes can be counted, sometimes aiding in diagnosis of other malformations that fit in with a suspected disorder suggested by a family's history. Fetal blood diseases (e.g., sickle cell disease, beta-thalassemia, hemophilia) are among those that can be diagnosed with this technique. A recent advance was made for diagnosis of sickle cell disease by studying DNA of fetal cells, which might make fetoscopy unnecessary for this disorder. Fetoscopy has a higher risk of fetal death than amniocentesis, perhaps between 3 and 4 percent.

Ultrasound is a technique whereby high frequency, low intensity sound waves are directed through the mother's abdomen via a transmitter. The same transmitter receives the returning signals reflected from the fetus. These are transposed visually onto a screen. Ultrasound machines are used in tandem with amniocentesis and fetoscopy, both to assure the position of the fetus and to guide the physician. Also, ultrasound is used to assess fetal age and to diagnose problems with the fetal skull, body, or intestinal tract. There are no known risks related to sonography.

The future of prenatal diagnosis may lie in studies of fetal cells retrieved from the mother's blood as early as ten weeks into gestation. Not only can these be obtained at a much earlier date than is safe to use amniocentesis, but the risks of a needle puncture may be altogether avoided. Herzenberg and colleagues have developed a cell-sorting machine, which enables different kinds of cells to be separated from one another after being stained with a preparation that makes them fluorescent.[10]

Parents get good news about 96 percent of the time following prenatal diagnosis, in that the disease or defect that was suspected is not present in the fetus. In the remaining 4 percent, the collected experience of most physicians is that parents choose abortion with few exceptions. Perhaps this means that most parents already have their minds made up about the abortion issue before starting prenatal diagnosis. There are a few reported cases of parents requesting prenatal diagnosis with a position against abortion and not changing their minds after learning a serious disorder is present.[11]

Can Genetic Disorders and Congenital Malformations Be Treated?

Therapy, including surgery, for the newborn with a genetic disorder or serious malformation has been possible in the past. Dietary measures, vitamin therapy, surgery for cleft lip and palate, and the many surgical and medical steps needed to treat spina bifida are only a few examples. In the past, treatment of the developing fetus has been mainly restricted to those that will be affected by the mother's sensitization to Rh factor if not treated with gamma globulin or by transfusion.

The public can expect to hear much more about fetal therapy, because physicians and scientists are both learning more about the opportunities to treat disease prenatally and conducting more clinical trials. The use of ultrasound as a method of detection of disorders or developing malformations is a main source of these new opportunities. Unless the affected fetus can be helped, in many instances, continued growth would mean a progressively worse outcome. For example, physicians in California recently operated successfully to relieve the results of congenital hydronephrosis in the growing male twin of a female fetus.[12] In this disorder, a congenital defect prevents the normal growth of the ureter that empties the fetal bladder and urine is obstructed, which can lead to serious prenatal brain damage. By inserting a catheter through the mother's uterus into the affected area in the fetus, the blocked urine is drained. More surgery follows after birth to correct the problem in a more definitive way. The twins and their mother are doing well today.

The same group of fetal surgeons more recently removed a twenty-one-week-old fetus from the uterus, repaired congenital defects in both ureters, and returned the fetus to the womb to complete gestation.[13] The fetus survived the surgery and the mother completed pregnancy; she gave birth by Caesarean section with no complications to her. Unfortunately, previous damage done by the disease was so extensive to the lungs, bladder, and kidneys of the infant boy that, after nine hours of mechanical support in the neonatal intensive care unit, he was allowed to die.

The majority of treatments available are now done in cases where the problem would be diagnosed early with ultrasound and an early delivery planned, concurrent with surgery or other treatment, in order to help the infant. Sometimes an early Caesarean delivery is preferable, as for example when the fetus is developing hydrocephalus (an enlarged head caused by too much fluid in the normal fluid spaces in the brain).

Some of the most interesting research in the near future should uncover ways to treat the fetus for some of the most devastating causes of harm to human life, such as nutritional deficiency and growth retardation. These possibilities, along with others on the cutting edge of fetal therapy, were reviewed in a 1981 medical article along with the unique ethical issues that will accompany fetal therapy.[14]

The ultimate type of genetic therapy would be to correct the problem at the root cause—namely, to replace a gene or genes sending incorrect messages with DNA prepared by humans in a laboratory that corrected the message or to replace the faulty genes altogether. There is a great deal of current interest in the use of genes "purified" in the laboratory, using new techniques of recombining DNA, and the use of these genes as therapeutic agents in humans. Experiments with animals, especially the mouse, are underway that should tell us if these techniques (1) work, and (2) cause no harm to the offspring for several generations. It is too early to hope for gene therapy in humans until more evidence from animal experiments is done. We must all be reminded how necessary it is to protect patients in medical research and how much depends on the conscience of physicians to protect people from the risks of research. Clergy are expected not only to help the users of applied human genetics to find their way through difficult decisions, but to be aware of a researcher's temptation to abuse the rules and guidelines that regulate research. Which clergyperson knows when he or she might be consulted by a gifted scientist whose new idea may be valid but premature? Case 5 illustrates this problem.

Case 5. Attempted Gene Therapy[15]

In May 1979, Dr. Martin Cline, a physician-scientist at UCLA, sent a proposal to a review committee of the institution to treat patients with sickle cell disease and other diseases of hemoglobin. Among the experimental treatments proposed was one using recombinant DNA. His plan was to use "purified" genes, made in the laboratory, that copy the correct message for the function that is missing and insert them in the bone marrow of sick patients. Dr. Cline's colleagues on the review committee, persuaded by consultants that more animal experiments were needed, voted in July 1979 not to recommend the plan.

Dr. Cline travelled to Europe in June, before the review group's decision. He took with him samples of human globin genes that he had prepared in his UCLA lab using funds from, among others, NIH. He intended both to do laboratory experiments with the DNA (to see if the lab-prepared DNA would grow in bone marrow) and to do a clinical trial with patients in Israel and Italy. Dr. Cline contacted physicians in Israel and Italy to help him with these experiments and to locate suitable patients.

The hospital in Israel, a part of the Hadassah Medical Center, required that a review committee similar to the UCLA group pass on the experiment. The Israeli committee inquired in the United States to make sure that rules for using recombinant DNA were clear to them. Dr. Cline informed the Israeli group that the experiment did not involve DNA fragments that would be prohibited from use in the United States by NIH rules. The experiment was approved. He then proceeded to use recombinant genes in attempting to insert betaglobin genes in the bone marrow of a twenty-one-

year-old woman with beta-thalassemia, a disorder of the hemoglobin for which there has been no treatment other than repeated transfusion. (The transfusions harbor dangers of their own: most
beta-thalassemia patients die from iron overload.) In Naples, he
later attempted the same treatment on a sixteen-year-old girl with
the same disorder. Written informed consent was obtained in both
cases. After his return to the United States, a storm of objections
rained down from fellow scientists. No change was reported in the
patients as a result of the experiment.

In 1981, following an official inquiry by NIH, it was found that
Dr. Cline had substantially violated safeguards of human subjects in
research. He subsequently resigned his chairmanship of a department at UCLA but remained on the faculty and medical staff. In
any subsequent application for federal support of his research, the
report of the inquiry into his attempted gene therapy will be attached. Dr. Cline explained that his decision to treat the patients
with recombinant DNA was made "on medical grounds," but that
he greatly regretted his "decision to proceed with the use of recombinant molecules without first obtaining permission from the appropriate committees." (The prospect for gene therapy in humans is
discussed in the final chapter.)

2. Ministry as Faithful Companionship

I hope that this book will be used by clergy, especially by those who work in congregations, hospitals, and counseling centers. I also hope that it will be used by laity who will be parents or who already have a reason to be concerned about their risks of reproduction.

Of almost 500,000 clergy in the United States,[1] the majority, over 300,000, serve in congregations of at least 219 different religious bodies. The theological and ethical concepts that form these many traditions are diverse. The cultures that these groups transplanted to the United States, along with their religious expressions, are also many-splendored. In the midst of this variety of religion and culture are great differences of opinion concerning the role of an ordained leader, a member of the clergy. Concepts of ministry, priesthood, rabbinate, and spiritual guidance are quite different. Rabbis are expected to be expert scholars of Jewish tradition and literature, in addition to performing many other liturgical and community leadership responsibilities. Priests of Roman Catholic, Orthodox, and parts of the Anglican traditions are expected to be sacramental and liturgical leaders. Protestant churches vary widely in their expectations of clergy, but perhaps stress most the tasks of preaching and Biblical teaching.

The question, "What ought clergy be and do?" is likely never to be answered by consensus. Are differences between religious bodies so great as to defeat any effort to communicate across them, especially about what ministry means? I have an intuition, nurtured by experiences in interfaith theological education and supported by some recent research, that despite real theological differences about the role and authority of religious leaders, there is a concept or model of ministry that can be shared by most clergy. Namely, clergy are expected to be faithful companions in times when religious need is greatest—that is, when people are in the stress and anxiety of a crisis. This role is one among many, but it is one that is assumed by clergy of every religious body.

Social scientists and leaders in theological education recently concluded a major study of the question, "What are the similarities and differences that members and clergy of 47 denominations have in their expectations of what a seminary graduate should be and do?"[2] The study involved the issue of *readiness* for ministry rather than what a seasoned veteran looks like twenty years later. Theological educators often ask themselves, "What is the role for which we are educating our students?" Seminary officials know that they may, for theological or ethical reasons, decide to educate students differently than the prevailing view about what a seminary graduate should be able to do. But they decided that good research on expectations ought to be done.

The most striking finding is the importance of the *person* of the ordained religious leader and the authenticity of his or her faith. A lower importance is placed on the ecclesiastical or social activities of the clergy. In short, American religious bodies appear to expect the clergy to be persons of integrity willing to serve without much acclaim. The most desirable characteristics that clergy should have, in the view of these respondents, is to lead openly and responsibly. They should have their heads and hearts together in the times they are most needed: when people are in stress. American religious bodies do not tolerate unethical or dominating behavior and undisciplined living in their leaders. They will not long condone self-servingness or withdrawal from the seas of troubles in which people find themselves. The respondents were largely not high on ecclesiastical or social advocacy of clergy. But my experience tells me that the clergy's community activities or advocacy of unpopular causes will be tolerated or even appreciated if those clergy are also consistently faithful companions in times of great trouble or joy.

My intuition is also based on several years' experience in organizing the education of seminarians in the context of congregations. These students served in congregations of their own denominations, bodies that spanned the Protestant, Jewish, and (to a lesser extent) Catholic families of religious traditions. We experimented with many forms of evaluation of the work of the students, as well as their clergy supervisors. We learned firsthand the rich differences in expectations of a rabbi, pastor, and priest. However, one theme of ministry linked diverse expectations of clergy and theological students. This theme of ministry is inherent in the question, "Is he or she *really* there when you are in need?" I emphasize the word "really" to point out that clergy are expected to be *real* or authentic in the times when only a religious leader can provide the kind of help that is needed. These times of deepest religious need are when persons are most aware of their limits, fragility, and potential as human beings. It is at these times that they most need a faithful companion.

The Human Need for Religious Guidance

Religion, in my view, is a process for making sense in ourselves when conflicts that arise from the condition of being human threaten to tear apart our basic confidence that we are worthwhile. Everyone engages in religion who seeks help or gives it when the vital core of confidence in the meaning of life is threatened. Only human beings can symbolize what affirms or threatens the fragile tissue of basic confidence that "the whole business of living," as it were, is irreducibly good. Without a sense of trust in being at all, what Paul Tillich called "the courage to be," the root of the vine of human life withers and dies. There is in human beings a need and a capacity for responding to the need for reassurance that all is well at the heart of the matter of living. The symbolic ship in us that houses that basic confidence is the something in us that must be moored to the bank. Many things happen in the story of a human life that threaten to dislodge the ship permanently. In these times of crisis, religious guidance is most needed.

Let us move from the basic meaning of religion to a more general consideration of the need for religious guidance. I have long been impressed with the similarity between the process of religious crises in later life and that which Erik Erikson described as the first and fundamental crisis of human life, whether "basic trust" will be a reality in the life of the new infant.[3] The infant, so recently secure and enveloped in warmth, is frightened and hungry. Basic trust in the child is the sense of optimism encouraged by the fact that "somebody is there," namely, the mother *and* the somebody in the child who needs the mother and responds to her. If there is something wrong at either end of this original reciprocity, both mother and child will suffer, but the child will die mentally. Some infants die physically if deprived of the mother's or another's warmth, body, and closeness. Are not the simplest dynamics of religion at work in the infant's need not to feel hungry, abandoned, and threatened, when just a little while before all was well? The disturbed infant feels the mother's secure arms, eats and is calmed. When the infant can see her face and be recognized in turn, the sense of basic trust is deepened by tender interchanges of mother and child. For better or worse, our parents are our first companions in life. Apparently, human beings are born with the need to feel basically secure and the ability to respond in a process designed to meet this need.

The problem, due to the condition of being human, is that it is never the lot of humans to be secure. Conflicts and threats from within and without continue to disturb the original sense that everything is or will be all right. The child sees death portrayed on television. A favorite pet is run over in the street. Baby sister dies. When a child becomes aware of death is an interesting issue, but not nearly as interesting as *that* a child becomes aware of death. Self-awareness and death-awareness are the distinctly human characteristics, but these very marks of being human are great sources of anxiety and terror. Beginning with the threat of death, which is the supreme threat to any confidence that living is worthwhile, life poses a long series of terrors to individuals and their culture.

Because we are born "unfinished" to a remarkable degree, as compared to other species, the human world is more open than closed. A mouse's world is circumscribed by instinct modified by training. The human world is open in the sense that it can both be imagined differently and modified beyond the limit of any previous arrangement that helps us to navigate that world. The quality of freedom in the human ability to respond to many things and many sources of action is the condition of being human. But there is a price for using freedom and being in it. Human beings feel anxious because nothing in their world is really closed. The basic purpose of culture and society, as described so well by Peter Berger,[4] is to bring enough closure and order to freedom for human activities to proceed.

The argument thus far is that there is a need for religious guidance in every human being and in every human collective with a distinct identity to maintain in time. Beyond the primal security evoked by the mother and child, other social relationships must replace the indispensable work that began between them. Religious institutions provide the patterns of guidance that continue to redirect anxiety about existence towards sources of reassurance. But I hasten to add that the process that is so obvious in religious institutions is not confined to them.

The process of religion is universal and ubiquitous. In every sphere of human life and institutions I see people hard at work trying to make enough sense out of apparent nonsense to restore enough confidence to remain loyal to difficult tasks. Religious work is quite visible when people involved in a particular enterprise stop to remember who they are, what their responsibilities are, and where they are going. In the family reunion, the elders tell the younger members about times when the future of the family was threatened and how certain qualities saw them through disaster. In the convocation, the leader of the institution tells the assembled members what the problems are, the threats to the integrity of their cause, and how the threats can be overcome. When a new head of state is chosen, the ceremony usually involves reflections on the past and destiny of the nation, sometimes devolving upon the poet to tell. Between the lines of stories, exhortations, and verse emerges the outlines of the desperate human struggle to be and remain sane in the midst of a world, in the words of Ernest Becker, where "each thing, in order to deliciously expand, is forever gobbling up others."[5] The need for religious guidance is everywhere shared by all. In the religious institutions, however, patterns of religious guidance evolved to their finest point. The religious leader is expected to be a faithful companion *par excellence* to those whose basic confidence in the worth of "the whole business" has been shaken or torn apart.

What Does It Mean to Be a Faithful Companion?

The word "companion" can mean many things. Three familiar meanings are comrade, one who accompanies another, or one who is employed to live with and serve another. The roots of the word are twofold. *Com* (from the Latin *cum*, or with) and *panis*, the Latin word for bread. A companion is one who is with you with bread.

The symbolism of bread is rich and varied. The daily meal with companions and the sacramental meal come to mind. We need daily bread to live, and the Gospels (Matt. 4:4, Luke 4:4) express the teaching of Jesus that humans need something more than food for life. Jesus described our dependence on "every word that proceeds from the mouth of God." The symbol of bread as word of God connects with the discussion of religion in the previous section. Without an unshakable confidence that life is worthwhile, even the will to make bread and eat it is threatened. Jesus' teaching, in concert with the Hebrew prophets, points to the radical human dependence on a power outside ourselves as the source of this confidence. The word most often used in religious traditions to describe the relation between God and humans is "faith."

The Latin word from which "faith" is translated is *fides. Fides* is better understood as "trust" than as a series of doctrines or articles in a creed. The link between *fides* and the word translated "confidence" should be clear. A study of the meanings of the word "faith" requires tracing the links between three words: faith, Amen, and sin.[6]

The Hebrew word for faith, *emunah,* is derived from a root, *amin,* that means "to be firm or sure." The utterance *Amen* is derived from the same root. Amen, uttered in Hebrew and Aramaic at the end of prayers, conveys agreement with the reliability of God and an intention to carry out a vow. In the New Testament, Amen also conveys an answer of "yes" (Rev. 1:7, Rev. 22:20, 2 Cor. 1:20) to the reality of God who affirms the life of the believer with a prior "yes." The "yes" conveys that what God has done is reliable and true. Jesus' use of Amen in many places before his sayings is done to convey that the teachings are reliable and true. The Amen means, "this is the way life really is." The Gospels use the Amen in relation to Jesus' sayings thirty times in Matthew, thirteen times in Mark, six times in Luke, and twenty-five times in John, liturgically doubled.

The third word required to understand the meaning of faithfulness is its opposite, sinfulness. The root meaning of the verb in Hebrew and Greek that is translated "to sin" is the same in both languages. The secular meaning of the word in Hebrew means "missing the right point." Proverbs 19:2 expresses this meaning, by saying that the wayfarer that "hasteth with his feet sinneth" (i.e., goes astray). The root of the verb in Greek "to sin," *harmatano,* also means "to miss" or "not to hit," as in missing the point or not hitting the mark with one's response. The human responses that are, by contrast, sinful or unfaithful are evasion, sidestepping, or avoiding reality.

Religion is often portrayed as a fundamental avoidance of reality. Freud defined religion as an illusion. Marx decried religion as an "opiate of the people" used in the interest of the ruling class to soften the pain of the exploitation of the working class. I do not deny that participation in the religious process can be, and often is, filled with illusion and transparent maneuvers to mask injustice. My argument is that it is not necessary that illusion and injustice be presuppositions for participation in the religious process.

Religion does not necessarily mean denial of the terrors of living. Religion, as I have learned it, means needed help to face the full meaning and impact of every terror, especially death. On the other side of the experience of facing and learning about every terror, with the experience "behind" you, as it were, you discern that a power and strength not your own upheld you even when nothing else could hold your confidence together. If the principle for participation in the religious process is that there is no reality, except the reality of God, that cannot be fully known and faced, then nothing prevents us from challenging every illusion and injustice. I understand this to be the principle of monotheism.

The essential message of Jesus' teachings, as I have learned them, is at one with the monotheistic principle of the entire Bible. "There is none good but one," that is, God (Matt. 19:17). No other reality or power is to be treated with the ultimate respect that is due God. From this first principle, it follows that every other form of power is thereby relativized and encountered in a perspective in which nothing is to be feared or respected absolutely. Remaining loyal to the monotheistic principle, in spite of all terrors of life and death, is the goal of the religious process transmitted through Jesus and the Hebrew prophets.

Ministry as faithful companionship is the primary model of religious guidance that I have learned and which I try, with help, to practice. Religious guidance is needed to enable the religious process to reach its goal. My aim is to persuade you that this model of ministry is based on an understanding of religion that many people in this culture would find risky but eventually liberating.

Specifically, I see Jesus' teaching on the meaning of discipleship as true religious guidance to all who would follow him to learn the meaning of life without resort to illusion or injustice. I use the term "true" here not to exclude other forms of religious guidance. I do claim that his teaching illuminates human experience and can be borne out by our common experience. The teaching is "firm and sure," and is in this sense faithful and true.

The essence of Jesus' teaching on discipleship is found in the saying, "For whoever chooses to save his life will lose it, but who loses his life for my sake and the Gospel's will save it" (Mark 8:35, Matt. 10:39, Luke 17:33, John 12:25). The word in Greek translated by most Bible scholars "to save" stems from a root meaning "to preserve safe and unharmed." The word for savior, *soter*, comes from this same root. An ancient Hellenistic ruler was the *soter* of his people. He preserved the people and kept them from harm. The teaching is that, as long as we obey the desire to keep ourselves safe and unharmed, we lose our "lives." In the religious context, the word in the text translated into "life" is the Greek word normally pronounced *psyche* in English but better rendered *psyuche*. In other versions of Scripture, this word is also translated "soul." In modern English, "a whole, united self" comes closest to translating what *psyuche* means in its original form. The root of *psyuche* is the same as the root for the verb "to breathe," which is likewise the origin of the Hebrew word for spirit, *ruach*.

In using Jesus' saying in the Gospels, their authors addressed the possibility that martyrdom was a choice that some in the early churches would have to face. Some scholars suggest that the original saying of Jesus ran in perfect parallelism, "Whoever shall save his life shall lose it, but whoever shall lose his life shall save it," and Mark adds the words, "for my sake and the Gospel's" to press a point about the meaning of martyrdom.[7] However, martyrdom is only one terror. The consistency of the teaching holds true with all forms of threat to "the whole, united self." The meaning of life is found by taking risks with all forms of temporary security, not for our own sakes, but for the cause to which Jesus was loyal—that is, that God is the inexhaustible source of life and meaning. Paradoxically, it is by risking security that we find true security that withstands any threat.

To summarize, threats to the sense that human existence is supposed to make arise at all stages of life and in every quarter of society. These threats injure the emotional, ethical, and theological dimensions of the human self. Human beings have a need for reassurance of an original confidence that the goodness of life can be trusted. To help in the process by which that need can be addressed and met, we need faithful companions who will neither abandon themselves or others in the process. A faithful companion to others is one who is with them to help heal injuries to the core of the human ability to respond faithfully to the ultimate limits and potentials of being human. What the faithful companion has mostly to offer is the bread of reality and the symbolic bread of the word of God that can transform even the worst terrors of reality.

The Clergy as Faithful Companions

Although any person can act as faithful companion to others in the religious process, the clergy role has evolved into one of the most complex set of obligations and expectations for faithful companionship. Clergy, more than others, are expected to be present and work with those in great spiritual distress, who want and need their help, until some resolution occurs. Clergy are excused from the routine obligations of their everyday duties in such times, and no blame attaches to the long hours spent with families, individuals, or human groups on the brink of despair. For the clergy, this type

of companionship is only one part of a more extensive set of obligations. My argument is that it is so central to the clergy role that
members of different religious traditions can engage in the subject
matter of this book with emphasis on what unites the religious traditions.

How do we become and remain faithful companions? Obviously,
the clergy do not become faithful companions overnight, or simply
by thinking about it. The clergy stereotype, portrayed in cartoons
and films, is of a marginal, ineffectual person who observes the
struggles of life over the edge of a teacup or from the pulpit. As you
may suspect, I have not always held firmly or practiced the model
of ministry that I describe here, but with help from other faithful
companions, I make it my business to try.

My experience tells me that the standards of faithful companionship that are practiced in the congregations and families of the
clergy are the strongest determinants of what will or will not happen
between clergy and distressed persons in times of crisis. In short,
the religious process itself is the heart of the life of the congregation. Family process requires the religious process at vital points in
family history. In the beginnings of each new life the seeds of integrity in the self need to be nurtured. The religious process is so
closely linked to the family process that, much of the time, they are
interdependent. One way to measure the depth of need for religious
guidance in any society is the extent to which religious institutions
are required to add to and strengthen the religious process that
begins to function in the relationship of mother to child. In my
view, congregations can be best understood as training camps for
the struggles of life. Families are the primary groups from which we
gain or lose strength to respond creatively in the struggles to be and
remain human. Clergy spend most of their time in the essential
tasks of these two closely linked institutions. Congregations and
families have evolved the most complex set of roles and obligations
to enable participation in the religious process to meet its intended
goal, however transient the help may be.

If the clergy become real or authentic as religious leaders, there is
a higher probability that they will be accepted as faithful companions to those in great need. It is also vital that clergy be effective
members of their own families. It is highly unlikely that clergy who

avoid the risks of speaking to their own parents or spouse in a direct manner will be able to risk directness with others. One of the most significant problems of theological education is that, although a structure has evolved to help seminarians to learn the basic principles and content of the traditions, there is not yet a sufficient structure to help test their emotional, ethical, and theological capabilities of becoming leaders in congregations, not even to speak of being adequate members of families.[8]

The territory or "turf" that opens up in a crisis spans the emotional, ethical, and theological dimensions of the problem at hand. Clergy will feel confident to walk out on this turf without apologizing if they are already doing it in their congregations and families. If the religious process in the congregation or clergy family has atrophied, it is highly unlikely that clergy can be expected to function well in times of great stress. Their religious authenticity in the troughs of despair will be largely influenced by the degree of religious authenticity they have in the life of the congregation and family.

In working with groups of laity from different religious bodies prior to an experiment in theological education in the context of congregations, my colleagues and I asked them to describe major problems they had experienced with clergy over their lifetimes.[9] In more than twenty such group interviews, five problems consistently emerged with the same order of priority that foreshadowed the findings of the Readiness for Ministry study almost ten years later. We came to call the first problem "religious inauthenticity." The repeated comments of laity that evoked this category were: "he speaks down to us . . . did not have head and heart together . . . pious . . . hypocritical . . . lost on a mountaintop . . . did not live the gospel in his own life . . . treated the congregation like children . . . could not relate religion and life's problems. . . . There was also coherence on the other four problems: organizational ineffectiveness, personal problems, family problems, and financial problems. The strongest significance, however, was attached to the issue of religious authenticity.

How do religious leaders become authentic in their ministries? How does a person become a minister, priest, or rabbi in truth and not in name only? The clergy and the laity must take this step together. Clergy and laity must make the choice to be faithful companions to one another. Religious authenticity is conditioned upon whether clergy and laity face the terrors and threats to their basic confidence in their own relationships, and emerge stronger and more secure as a result.

My experience tells me, supported by such research that exists on the religious process in congregations,[10] that clergy and groups of lay persons go through critical stages in their relationships. These stages, which are the same as in the religious process in any other context, lead to moments of decision in which growth or retardation in the religious process is possible. Both laity and clergy have their own part to play in the precipitation and resolution of each crisis.* Three major crises can generally be observed: (1) testing the new clergyperson's authenticity; (2) playing God; and (3) developing particular authenticity.

Testing the New Clergyperson's Authenticity

The first crisis usually begins in the first or second year of service of a new clergyperson in the congregation. There is a well-known "honeymoon period" during the first few weeks or months of the new relationship. Everyone smiles and nods at first, but soon typical conflicts emerge. These are best described as "testing" the personal strength of the clergy and the capacity of the congregation to test the clergy (or any other newcomer for that matter). Congregations that have no tests for newcomers, no "cost of discipleship," cannot expect to exist long or thrive. Any time a newcomer enters a group with a distinct history, there will be testing. In congregations, testing can take the form of comparisons to the clergyperson's predecessor. Or there can be power struggles with leading laity about the clergy's right to change existing programs or priorities. The clergyperson feels that the congregation is watching closely, observing every mood and move. "Being sized up" is a common expression for this experience.

---

*However, I must observe that congregations generally hold the power to authenticate ("make real") the person and work of the clergy, even in denominations with hierarchical structures and episcopally defined ordination policies. Simply being ordained by a bishop is no guarantee of religious authenticity.

One can also easily observe nonsensical events in the new relationship of clergy and laity. Sermons ring out with bold statements about team ministry before there is any team. Clergy can also be seen to engage in some "crusade" in the first year, usually self-defeating. The new program may be totally inappropriate. Critical arguments are withheld. Laity watch passively while the new leader flounders.

The purpose of the testing is to discover if there is enough personal reality in the minister and congregation to lure them into any kind of deeper relationship in which the issues of power, authority, and ministry can be negotiated. The role of the congregation at this stage is to test the personal reality and integrity of the clergy. If members are too weak to test the newcomer, nothing of great significance can be learned or done with the disappointments of early hopes. The exaggerated idealism of their beginnings needs to be revised in the light of reality. If the realities of this early pain are avoided, growth is arrested. If the clergy do not pay attention to these early difficulties and try to avoid the pain by some early success-oriented project or program, a pattern of permanent avoidance can set in. Life in some congregations is dull and tepid, similar to a marriage that persists but does not live. This condition could be due to clergy and laity "keeping their lives safe" early in the relationship by turning away from the risks of facing the trouble towards something more comfortable but deadly.

Congregations and clergy arrested at this stage of the religious process show many signs of distress. The clergy expect too much too soon. The more anxious the clergy are about the deterioration of hopes, the more strident and complaining the message sent to the laity, although the message is veiled behind the rhetoric of lofty ideals. The message is, "You are disappointing me, you are not the zealous group you led me to believe you to be." The more hidden, angry messages that are sent by clergy to the congregation, the angrier the laity become, and they return a message (usually unspoken or said to third parties): "Are you for real? When are you going to grow up? We have other responsibilities rather than to work for the congregation fulltime!"

Nothing of significance happens to the troubled new relationship of clergy and laity until there is mutual recognition of the problem, and the problem can be discovered only if there is enough personal strength in the clergy and laity to pay attention, take risks, and ask for help. Often, it requires the help of other faithful companions to take this step. Laity who receive word from people in distress that the new clergyperson was of little help had best examine how they themselves might have contributed to the problem by avoiding trouble that they helped to make. Clergy who know that they are of little help in the first crises they try to meet had best examine what they are doing to lay the groundwork of faithful companionship in the fundamentals of their relationship to laity. Clergy who neglect to admit the need for laity as faithful companions can spin their wheels fruitlessly for years.

Clergy need to be reasonably known and trusted before they are "called" into the deeper life problems of the laity or before they can assume a helping role in the wider community. The religious language of "call" points to the difference between a compulsive response to cries for help and a considered response based on choice. The call of God is by definition answerable only by choice. Many clergy will remember that the first requests for pastoral help in a new congregation turned out to be from the most chronically depressed individuals or families. New clergy spend endless hours with such people, and some never wake to the fact that they are being used as well as using these cases to establish some early success. Such people often exploit the clergy's own instability in a new position.

In a crisis, laity will generally ask clergy to help only after the initial stage of their relationship has been successfully concluded. Pastoral help is chosen help. Clergy who begin to help in a crisis by asking the right person if help is truly wanted show signs of having successfully come through early problems in a congregation. Willingness to be turned down is a sign of strength. Further, asking the right person if help is wanted places the clergy in the position of being able to ask the other for help, which is always needed for the best outcome.

Playing God

The second crisis in the authentication of clergy begins around the issue of whether anyone is going to ask their help in the religious process. If no one invites, nothing happens. When people do begin to open doors and the clergy become credible companions in times of great trouble, the word spreads rapidly. As one Protestant minister put it, "crowds gather." People make their needs known without fear or hesitation. The word spreads to the community that the minister, priest, or rabbi is a real source of help. Some of the comments from laity who had found help from clergy were: "He is dedicated. . . . He had lived a full life and understood what I was going through. . . . He was a man of God and a man of the world. . . . He knew what to do when he visited my mother, because he was not afraid of death in the same way as the others and doctors. She died a peaceful death, much because the Reverend spent so much time with us and with her. . . . He is so open, and not embarrassed to express his feelings in public. I knew I could talk with him. . . ." These quotes emphasize personal integrity, openness, and religious commitment. Enough of these elements must be present for serious pastoral work to begin with persons who have been strong and well, but who are injured by the conflicts of living.

The second crisis appears to have three elements. First, it is precipitated by the clergy's attempts to meet a sea of human needs in the religious process. Great energy is required to provide religious guidance in crisis times. There is hardly any excitement to match that of moving into the deepest dilemmas and experiences of life with people who trust you and who want to learn to interpret their experience through the religious tradition that you represent. Calls increase from hospital, home, school, couples on the verge of divorce, successful people who worry about the price of success, and unsuccessful people who want to change. Needs deepen, people open up about their hunger for the way of discipleship. Closets with many skeletons are opened. Opportunities present themselves in every marriage, burial, and baptism to reconcile persons alienated by years of hatred, grudges, or guilty secrets. The experience of this work can be exhilarating. But it carries a heavy price.

Soon the situation begins to be oppressive. Laity with their eyes open can see the clergyperson deteriorating in front of them because of the burden of playing God. In worship, the sermon may be about the need to live dependently on God, but in reality the clergyperson acts as though he or she could meet any need. The crisis is one of professional authenticity in the deepest sense. The clergy, in the midst of self-imposed frenetic activity, do not practice in their lives what they preach by profession. The religious needs of the congregation are focused on the ordained leader who blindly tries to meet them all. Feeling that one can or must be a substitute for the religious process itself, clergy face a trap especially reserved for religious leaders. The symptoms of the clergy in this crisis are "the madness of God." Trying to play God, the all-giving Helper for others, leads to a desperate form of self-destruction. At the peak of the crisis, clergy accept call after call unthinkingly, often losing all track of time and concern for self, family, and peer relationships. Led on by the power to lead people onto holy ground, the clergy allow dependence to grow and feed on the appreciation of the crowds. All the while self-abuse increases. Many clergy have physical or emotional breakdowns during such crises in their careers, which often occur at the peak of what most would call "success." The despair that ensues from the corruption of the religious process itself is indeed profound. Many congregations suffer for years to come following the departure or untimely death of a religious leader in this situation.

Resolution of the crisis depends upon the capacity of laity to be faithful companions to the clergy, and if the clergy are willing to ask for and accept help. Laity who provide religious guidance for their religious leader are the backbone of a strong congregation. If they cannot do this task with confidence, the chances are slender that they could guide any newcomer or offer leadership to the community. The response of the clergy to the crisis of playing God is crucial. They can interpret it as a spiritual issue and openly share the dilemma, for they have substituted their work for their health, in the sense of *salus*. Laity who substitute work and career for the true meaning of life know the problem very well and can help convert the minister to a new way of living. The goal of the religious experience is the sincere acknowledgement of our total dependence on God. Not until the clergy's relationship to the congregation has the quality in it of living dependently on God, rather than the congregation's living dependently on the leader, is the crisis transcended.

Developing Particular Authenticity

After the experience of despair and new life generated by the second crisis, a period of harmony and well-being sets in. This, too, contains a critical turning point. I call it the crisis of particular authenticity, because the basic issue concerns the discovery of the clergyperson's own skills and capacities and how the work of the ministry will be shared. Recognizing that he or she cannot do all things well, and intensely sobered by the physical and emotional dangers of spiritual illusion, the clergyperson wants to share the ministry with other faithful companions. The laity, at this point, trust the clergyperson more and are motivated to share the work and honor his or her unique gifts.

This period is the best time for developing special interests and skills and collaborating with other professionals in the conduct of crises. Many clergy enter training programs or graduate work at the height of the first or second crisis, perhaps to avoid the risks of resolution. Laity who reflect on the clergy's intentions at such times correctly feel these moves to be avoidance. When the clergy have a secure base in the congregation because of the maturity and strength gained in the first few years, laity will gladly support and cooperate in a much more sophisticated approach to team ministry and interdisciplinary cooperation.

The approach that I take to the clergy's participation in the religious process as evoked in the context of bioethical dilemmas presupposes that the clergy have a deep base of support in their congregations and families for faithful companionship to those who practice applied human genetics or who use knowledge and techniques from these activities to make decisions about reproduction and parenthood. If this support is not present, the clergy will feel ill-equipped to tackle bioethics, and laity may feel neglected by a sudden, new interest when many fundamental problems of long-standing have not been resolved.

3. The Use of Genetic Information in Premarital Counseling

People who want to be married usually ask for the services of the clergy. In 1976, the last year for which statistics are available on numbers of marriages, eighty percent of the first marriages and sixty percent of the second or subsequent marriages in the United States took place in a religious setting.[1] There were in that year 1,706,628 marriages, of which 1,162,528 were first marriages for brides and grooms. Clergy were directly involved in 1,256,482 marriages in 1976.

The period prior to a marriage is rich with possibilities for faithful companionship to the couple and to their families in all branches. The religious process is vitally needed at this time by the families and the couple. If participation in the religious process is encouraged in a spirit of sincerity and truth (Josh. 24:14), the spiritual and physical health of the families and the couple can be enhanced. It is also a time when the clergy can help the couple to gather information relevant to their risks of reproduction, and refer them for genetic counseling.

Premarital Counseling

Virtually every denomination has requirements or customs that call for premarital counseling of the couple by the clergy. This counseling has several goals. First, there is a legal and public policy goal. Clergy are required in some states to be licensed by the jurisdiction in which they officiate as an officer of the state for solemnization of matrimony. The goal of the legal requirement is to make the officiant responsible, among others, for ascertaining that the laws of the state are not being violated by the marriage. These laws usually involve consanguinity (closely related persons), duress, age limitations, and compliance with blood tests to rule out venereal disease. Premarital counseling provides a greater opportunity to see the couple and thus rule out any legal barriers to the marriage. Many denominations have a minimal waiting period between the time the marriage is requested and its solemnization in a ceremony.

A historical note is appropriate on the background of the prevailing public policy on marriage. Marriage is seen, above all, as a voluntary activity in our society. We must not forget that marriage was not always voluntary, especially for children in families of some wealth or commercial standing. The poor have always had the benefits of "freedom of choice" in marriage. Prior to the sixteenth century in Western nations, most marriages were arranged by fathers. Great changes in marriage and family relations in the sixteenth and seventeenth centuries in European nations followed the Protestant Reformation.[2] The modern state and the nuclear family developed in the same cauldron of change. Gradually, the freedom of the individual to choose a marriage partner, to pursue self-fulfillment through marriage, and even to dissolve the marriage was increasingly enjoyed by all citizens. Patriarchal authority itself began to change with the spread of concepts of individual choice and egalitarianism. An ideal of marriage for love and companionship arose by the eighteenth century to replace the older community ideals behind patriarchal arrangement, although the economic function of marriage as the merger of the labor of two working households continued. Clergy are expected to officiate at marriages that are contracted in the spirit of a public policy that stresses the principles of freedom and fairness in the relations between the sexes.

A second goal of premarital counseling is to help the couple test their personal strength and maturity to carry out the obligations of marriage. A third goal concerns teaching the couple, if needed, the special emphasis of the religious tradition of the officiant as to marriage and possibly divorce. Some denominations have modest to severe restrictions on a person who requests marriage after divorce. In a pluralistic society with so many religious bodies, premarital counseling is also a setting for exploration of the religious preferences of the couple. If the couple are from very different denominational backgrounds, they may decide to unite their preferences in one religious body; or they may remain in their respective denominations with a clearer picture of the differences and similarities.

For the first ten years of my pastoral service, I practiced premarital counseling largely in terms of the second and third goals. I conducted an "exercise in listening" as the couple told me about their relationship, its strengths and weaknesses, and I helped them identify problems for which they might need more help. I required at least two meetings. The first concerned the couple's expectations of marriage and experiences prior to marriage. If no outstanding barriers emerged in the first meeting, in the second meeting we worked through the text of the marriage rite and its vows as a structure for discussing the theological and ethical meaning of marriage.

In the first meeting, I tried to make the couple comfortable, because they would come both not knowing what to expect and also secretly expecting that my role was to make them confess to me what their sexual experience had been prior to marriage. I usually opened the meeting by saying that they had a choice about the agenda of these premarital counseling meetings. They could use them to explore with me, in confidence, the strengths and weaknesses of their relationship to date. If, after considering whether they chose to talk to me "personally" about their relationship, they decided against it, we could then proceed to study the meaning of marriage, and to plan the service, by reviewing the contents of the marriage rite. I cannot remember one couple in those years that turned down the opportunity to talk about their relationship. In this period (1956 to 1966), I officiated in approximately fifty weddings.

My memory of the premarital counseling I did in these years is of pleasant, conventional talks with earnest couples about their aspirations and plans. The most serious troubles with which I dealt concerned marriage after divorce. During and following the weddings that I conducted in these years, I noticed that everyone appeared happy except me. I expected to be fufilled by helping young couples in such moments but, to the contrary, I was depressed and lonely. I recall feeling lonely in the wedding receptions I attended as the officiant. I was spoken to politely, but essentially as a functionary. I was always eager to leave as soon as possible. Reflecting on those years, I indeed fulfilled the clergy stereotype, passively observing the struggles of life over the edge of my eyeglasses in the "nondirective" mode of counseling, or over a champagne glass (rather than a teacup), as befits a good Episcopal clergyman.

I finally sought professional help for my feelings of depression and loneliness. I learned that one of the major reasons for my condition, in addition to other causes, was that I was not doing the job that clergy are expected to do at such crucial times. Curiously, I felt that the couple were doing me and my congregation a favor by asking for the wedding, rather than our giving them a serious opportunity for both families to participate in a religious process. I held standards about marriage and adult relationships about which I was silent even as I saw the couple and their parents violating them during the premarriage period. I listened to them tell me about unresolved problems with their parents that ranged from old grudges and concern about a parent's alcoholism, to their awareness of serious parental objection to their marriage. I squelched my need to be responsible in the face of these and other issues, mainly in the interest (I now believe) of avoiding the hard work of tackling matters of responsibility in my congregations and family. I did not use the authority that my church had invested in me to set an example of "sincerity and truth" for the couple and families. Out of these painful discoveries about my avoidance of the hard work of being an effective minister, I began to forge some new standards for these and other encounters.

Premarital Counseling and the Religious Process

The social and religious significance of marriage is caught up in the biblical text, "Therefore shall a man leave his father and mother and shall cleave unto his wife, and they shall be one flesh" (Gen.

2:24). Nowadays, we must surely add (at least mentally) a man *and* a woman to the masculine reference in the text.

The basic problem of the premarital period is the abundance of nonsense that fills the air to contradict the most common assumptions about the institution of marriage. The couple are supposed to leave their parents and "forsake" all others. "Everybody knows" that the new husband and wife are supposed to begin a new relationship by leaving their parents and other lovers to make a new household. The obligations in the roles of husband and wife as embodied in the marriage vows assume that they are adults whose best interests are in keeping the promises. Presumably, the couple can now stand in the parental roles of those that they "leave" (i.e., they are social equals to their parents). Further, the couple is supposed to have left all previous intimate relationships with other males and females who have been competitors for the role of spouse now to be enjoyed by only one other. In my experience, it is rare that prior to marriage a young couple have completely untangled the webs of unfinished business with former lovers and the aspects of their relations with parents that can be brought to some closure.

The problem of "forsaking all others" can be greatly intensified if there has been a previous marriage that ended in divorce. If it is a first marriage, and the couple have had intimate experiences with others, or if one or both have lived with another person for a period, the clergy can observe firsthand the problems posed by the live strands of the previous relationships that persist and intrude upon the assumption that *only* these two persons are involved in marriage. The word "troth," from which the service of betrothal is taken, stems from a root in Old English meaning "truth." When the vows are taken, the expectation is that the couple is speaking the truth. Yet I have seen marriages begin more in a spirit of punishment of a former lover or spouse who abandoned the bride or groom than in a spirit of freedom and truth in the couples' choice of one another.

To complicate the matter, the vast majority of first marriage partners do not see themselves as equals of their parents, and most parents do not treat the new husband and wife as equals. The communication and behavior in the typical prelude to marriage is marked by parent-child rather than adult-to-adult characteristics.

For example, what looks like a simple matter—who first calls or contacts the clergy to ask for help with the marriage plans and service—turns out to be not so simple if a parent calls and says, "We want you to officiate at our daughter's (or son's) wedding." Does it make sense for a parent to make this request for those supposed to be responsible enough to vow "to love and to cherish until we are parted by death"? Does the couple really want their parents to handle their important responsibilities for them all of their lives? And do any rational parents really plan to take care of their children forever? The clergy, including myself, who allow the relationship to begin on the wrong premise may never get it back on the right premise.

The spirit of the initial contact for a future marriage can set a priority for companionship or polite social distance for the future relation of clergy, couple, and families. Why do they call for a religious leader at this time? The clergy can fall into the trap of believing that people want a religious ceremony because social convention requires it. This narrow view obscures the driving need for reassurance that humans feel as they enter the adult obligations that marriage entails and as they choose only *one* other to begin a relationship designed to succeed and even outstrip the parent-child arrangement. How do they know that they have chosen the *right* person? More deeply, have they "left" all of the others they might have chosen? The basic issue of the premarital period is: "Who am I now? How do I respond to the need to leave and also to the need to hold onto old arrangements that have brought me this far?" This is the issue for the couple and also for their parents, who need to let go of the past and begin to leave their children free to begin a new step of life with spouse and family.

The religious process is designed to enable the limits and possibilities of human experience of *separation* and *new beginnings* to be symbolized. Further, clergy can encourage participation in the religious process by modeling, with their own behavior, what faithful companionship entails.

To return to the not-so-simple problem of who first calls to make the marriage arrangements, let us suppose that it is a parent. The parent has, by calling, already decided to avoid having the couple call themselves. In addition, the parent takes over the couple's freedom to choose where, when, and by whom they want to be married. The clergy can begin the test then and there. One way of responding is, "I'm interested to hear about it, but I really prefer to be contacted by the couple themselves." Other ways of responding, perhaps more to the point are: "Did they ask you to call me?" or "Why are *you* calling me?" The immediate reaction of the parent may be bristling irritation, but you can decide not to let the temporary security of being popular with the parent interfere with the job of being a good companion to both couple and parents. If more is needed by the parents to remind them that they are off-target, simply ask if they plan to be doing things like this for the rest of their lives. The parents usually get the point and make haste to have the couple call.

The initiation of premarital counseling begins with the first contact. If one of the couple calls me, after the introductory request, I usually ask if the other member of the couple is present. If so, I ask them both to speak to me by telephone or go to a place where two telephones are available. If the other is not physically present, or in another city, if at all possible I ask the caller to make arrangements for a three-way conference call. The first test should be about the conditions for beginning the premarital counseling relationship. If they have been accustomed to always having their way or to clergy rushing to help without asking any questions, perhaps this is an arrangement that needs to be left behind. More important, the couple should be treated as equals in requesting help to get married.

Usually the initial request is not for help, but, "We would like to get married. Would you do the ceremony?" They do not realize that the question does not logically follow the first statement. There is no necessary connection between my willingness to do the ceremony and their wish to get married. I usually say something like, "Wait a minute. Let's start over. Are you asking for my help in getting married?" If they say they are, or that such was their intention, I put them in a position of literally saying the words, "I want your help in getting married." If one of the couple says "we" rather than "I," I point out that my understanding is that he or she is not married yet and there is still time for a change of mind. Sometimes humor also helps to get a point across.

My goal in the first contact is that, at its conclusion, I will have taken the initiative in setting the terms of the relationship between the couple and myself to my satisfaction and also have given them a sufficient picture of the requirements of premarital counseling so that they can begin to work before the first meeting. If the request is to marry within a time frame of less than six weeks, I do not accept the assignment. I say simply that I have found it impossible to complete the work required in such a short time.

Before the initial contact is over, I clarify the fact that I am not agreeing to do the wedding, but only to a first meeting in which the necessary work will be explained more fully. I say that there are two requirements of my counseling. The first is that they be willing to work directly with parents or other relatives on family problems that need attention prior to the wedding. The second is that they will do some research in their families' health history and consult a qualified genetic counselor, usually a physician, with the results.

If they agree to these ideas, I then set a time for the first meeting and give them an assignment that I explain will be the subject of our first meeting. The instructions are: "By way of preparation for our meeting, I would like you to recall, and write down, if needed, those traditions and values in your family of which you are most proud and want to continue in your new family. Also, I want you to do the opposite. Are there any practices or customs that you consider harmful, and which you do not want to continue?" I explain that traditions and practices include everything from ways of celebrating holidays to ways of settling arguments. With their acceptance of the assignment, we agree to meet at the arranged time.

In the fourteen years since I began to change my practices of premarital counseling, I have been contacted by twenty-one couples with marriage plans. During those years I have been a seminary teacher, administrator, and bioethicist, which are not ideal positions for attracting large numbers of couples who want to be married. Six of these couples were in too great a hurry to accept my conditions. Fifteen couples did consult me about their plans, having asked for my help. In three of these cases, I was "fired" as the officiant-to-be, because their refusal to comply with the first requirement presented problems too great for me to continue. I have never been refused on the requirement of research on family health history.

Standards of Premarital Counseling

In the first meeting, I cover the two basic requirements for a second time. The telephone is not a perfect instrument. I also repeat that my understanding is that they have asked for my help in the tasks of preparing for marriage as well as, if I agree, my help to plan and perform a ceremony. I encourage them to tell me whatever is on their minds, especially if there is anything left over from our telephone discussions.

As I discuss the first requirement, I stress that adults are expected to speak to one another directly, without going through third parties, especially with important requests and feelings. If the initial contact came from a parent or only one of the couple, I return to the example to show why I insisted on speaking with both members of the couple before proceeding. I state that I assume that we will continue to practice the same standard, and if they see me breaking the standard, I need their help in reminding me of my responsibility. I point out further that I need their help in several ways to do my job as a minister with them and their families before and during the wedding ceremony. Specifically, I need their help to improve communication. If they bring up problems or feelings to me about their parents, other members of the family, former intimates, or former spouses, and it appears indicated that they should speak directly to these people about these problems, I ask them to do so if they agree that it is in their interest. I will not coerce them to do something that they decide is against their best interests.

My rationale for this standard is twofold. First, families thrive on direct communication of thoughts and feelings and tend to become troubled and even pathological if communication is indirect or through third parties. Second, I explain that the origin of the word "troth" is truth, and that when I am at the altar with them, I will feel better about myself and them knowing that we had left no stone unturned to clear the path to their future of as many obstacles as possible. At any rate, we are going to pray together during the wedding service. The prayers can either be a caricature of what prayer is supposed to be or be close to the truth. I define prayer as speaking directly, from the heart, to God about our needs. I observe that I have not known people who could pray authentically who also had difficulty speaking directly to other people about their needs.

As I close the description of the first requirement, I take a brief biographical history of each person. The history includes full name, date and place of birth, full name of parents and dates of birth, marital history of the couple and their parents, educational and work history of the couple and their parents, and religious history of the couple and their parents. The latter category includes facts about baptism, confirmation, and periods of activity and inactivity. The history is for my own records and to complete records required by the denomination. Additionally, the history gives me an opportunity to test the couples' impressions of pertinent facts about themselves and their respective parents.

I then review the second standard and my rationale for requiring them to do research on their own and their families' health history. I share with them the Family Health History Chart (Appendix C) as a way to structure the discussion. Working with the chart, the couple should be able to account for any significant genetic disease, mental retardation, and the cause of death for each close relative back to their grandparents. Unless they already know a physician or genetic counselor to whom to take the results of the homework, I am ready with a referral to one or more physician-geneticists with whom I regularly work.

I place three expectations on them: (1) they must do the work to complete the chart; (2) they must consult a qualified physician or counselor with the results who can answer questions about reproductive risks and family planning concepts; and (3) they will face up to the consequences of the information if it contains any bad news. If the inquiry shows that there are no known causes for worry, then we can proceed to other work. If, on the other hand, there are reproductive risks, these must be thoroughly discussed, along with their feelings about making the discovery.

Normally, I receive some resistance from the couple about seeking genetic information. "Why should we do that?" they sometimes ask. "You are not a physician." I explain that it is a precaution and insurance against an unknown risk that would tragically affect them and their children. If such happened and we had a chance to prevent it, and I knowingly walked to the altar with them without pointing out this chance, I would be part of the chain of events that led to their child's harm. I explain to them that I like to sleep at night and do not want such an event on my conscience. I also point out a possible higher risk of psychosocial distress and divorce among couples who have a child with a serious genetic disease.[3] In my experience, it is much more difficult for couples to carry out the first requirement than the second. They have much more resistance to facing the problems in their relationship to parents than the risks of reproduction.

If the couple agree to both standards, I then structure the next part of the meeting by asking them to go over the results of their reflections on the values and disvalues of their family traditions and practices. These discussions are rich opportunities to learn how much insight couples have into their respective families strengths and weaknesses. We then explore ways they can express gratitude for the former and act to correct the latter, if only to declare their awareness of the weaknesses and their consequences. The following cases, which are disguised, illustrate these opportunities.

Case 6: For Better or for Worse

A twenty-eight-year-old man, Jim, declared that he was proudest of his family's sense of "solidarity and continuity." Generations of his family members were close, according to him, having returned to the deep Southern family homestead for reunions and events such as his wedding-to-be. He was least proud of his father's practice of long-suffering and enduring humiliations by his mother, who was overbearing and selfish. His fiancée's parents had both died and Jim's parents had offered their home for the wedding, but now his mother was trying to take over all the arrangements for the wedding. He had recently hung up on her as she harangued him about the choice of dresses for the bridesmaids and other matters, telling him that he had to see to it that "those boys who are groomsmen have to have haircuts." When I asked Jim if he had communicated how he really felt about this to his father and mother to his satisfaction, he replied that he had tried, nothing had changed, and he was not satisfied. I asked his fiancée, Jane, if she had seen him express himself to his parents. She replied that she had. I asked her if he was effective and convincing. "About as convincing as a sniveling child," she answered with some vindictiveness in her voice and a near sneer on her face.

I then asked Jim if Jane had done anything yet to help him with his problem. He answered in the negative. I asked him, "Are you proud of her for standing by quietly while you flounder? I thought wives were supposed to help husbands. It says something in the vows about "for better or for worse, and so on." Jim replied to me that he was not proud of Jane. I asked him to tell her that directly, and to tell her as well, if he agreed, that spite was a poor substitute for help in getting a marriage off the ground. He exploded at her, "I am not proud of you! You are always treating me with contempt!" And he brought up other matters of long-standing.

Jane also had a chance to have her say about Jim. She brought up things she did not admire that went back to the beginning of their relationship, as well as the qualities that she did. She observed, with remarkable insight, that Jim was very like his father. He observed in return, and with some amazement, that Jane was like his mother. He marveled, "I read about it in books, but I didn't believe it." I pointed out to them that some experts on family process show how practices and patterns of avoidance are sources of trouble to families for generations, until someone who will take risks insists on a change.[4] Apparently, as we grow up in families, we inherit more than just eye and hair color. I asked them both how they felt so far, and they said they felt good.

I told them that before the next meeting, if there was to be one, I wanted to hear about how they had worked together to help Jim get the task done to his satisfaction and get some better treatment for himself. Jane protested, "But we've already had the invitations printed!" I commented that they could choose someone else if they really wanted to, but I could not conscientiously take a new step with them until they kept their end of the agreement. I asked them both if they felt it was in their best interests to take the step of helping one another. They agreed, looking reluctant, that it was in their best interest and that they would try. I said that I would not be happy with a "try." "Call me when you have *done* it," I said.

Jim called me some days later, alone and upset, saying that nothing had happened. Jane had refused to meet with his parents with him. She was urging him to "dump me" as the minister and find another one. According to Jim, Jane said, "We should just get through the ceremony as best we can and start our own life."

I told Jim that he and Jane should get on the phone together and fire me if that is the way they felt. Before that happened, however, I said that it was my duty to point out that if he could not count on her for this small task, what could he count on her for? And was not the fact that he was calling me all by himself making him look bad and reminding him of some other close relative? Was he really helping Jane by calling me on his own to complain about her? Is this the way a husband is supposed to help a wife? He was, I reminded him, supposed to call me with Jane when the job they were to do together, like married people, was done. There was a long silence at the other end.

"I am going to do this, or else," said Jim. I asked him to be sure what "or else" meant. He replied, "There are other women in the world." I asked him if he needed my help. He could call a family meeting anytime, if he chose to. If nobody came, he would at least know where he stood with a family proud of its "continuity and solidarity." He wanted to try it alone and would do it with or without Jane's help. I advised him to go to Jane, tell her of our discussion, and that they both should call me before seeing his parents.

A three-way telephone call enabled Jane to clear the air by telling me about her anger and resentment about my "catching her" in her lack of help to Jim. I said that she was entitled to be angry at me, just not entitled to let her husband down, which is what I tried to tell her. I asked Jim if he liked the way Jane was acting now with me. He said he did, that he felt she was being honest. This call ended with Jane and Jim making a plan to work together on communicating their feelings about Jim's mother's arrogance and mistreatment of Jim and his father. A family meeting ensued, initiated by the couple. This two-hour-long meeting ended with Jim inviting his mother to help him and Jane plan the wedding. At the rehearsal and ceremony, Jim's parents thanked me profusely for my help. The bride and groom were radiant.

Case 7: The Christmas Eve Snub

Widowed or divorced people who are being remarried often are aware of the bruised feelings of older children of the former marriage, who feel hurt by the proposed marriage and show their loyalty to the former spouse or envy of their parent's freedom. The following case illustrates this problem.

George and Jeanne, each once divorced, contacted me to request a wedding. Each former spouse was alive but not remarried. Jeanne had a family of three grown and married children, as well as two grandchildren. George had two children, one of whom was married, and no grandchildren. In the first meeting, Jeanne told of taking George to church on Christmas Eve to meet her oldest daughter and son-in-law, who left the church before the service ended to avoid any encounter. Angry phone calls followed. The bride wanted to pass off the experience; the groom was deeply offended but would not acknowledge it openly.

I recommended a meeting with all of the bride's children before proceeding any further, on the grounds that the children and the couple were acting in a manner that could diminish the chance that the marriage would succeed. I suggested strongly that both Jeanne and George be on the telephone together when they called Jeanne's children for a meeting. They agreed to take on this task and that it was in their best interest.

Later in the week, Jeanne called me to say dispiritedly that her daughter would not attend a meeting. I asked Jeanne two questions: "Do you have anything in your will about leaving her something?" She answered yes. "Have you learned anything in your career as a successful stockbroker that would help you with your daughter? You have clout with her, but you are not using it." I told Jeanne that without the meeting, I could not take a chance on going ahead.

Within an hour, I had a telephone call from Jeanne's daughter, saying that the meeting would be at her house. In a marathon three-hour meeting, each person had an opportunity to say what was on his or her mind. The main theme was the anger Jeanne's oldest daughter felt about her mother leaving her father. This daughter later boycotted the wedding, but at least she had cleared the air and given her mother an opportunity to listen and speak to her. Jeanne's other children did attend the wedding, along with the groom's children, and a follow-up showed that progress had been made in developing more honesty between the new couple and each of their children.

Case 8: Being Fired as the Clergy Consultant

At times, I have been "fired" by the couple who would not or could not accept the terms of the test I tried to give them. This case describes such a situation.

A couple (each once divorced) asked for my help in remarriage. Each had several grown children. A meeting was held with the woman's three children to discuss their family traditions and their feelings about their mother's plans. These children lived near their mother in the same city. Much progress was made, and the man appeared happy with his participation. He then spoke openly of his problems with two of his four children. However, when I suggested that a meeting was indicated with his children, he refused, shouting, "My problem with my daughter is ancient history and will not go away just because you want a meeting." I encouraged him to say more, but he refused. His wife-to-be could not change his mind, and he stormed out of the room. She called me later and said he would not speak to me. "I know what you are trying to do," she said, "but he can't do it right now." She stated that they would ask another minister to officiate. I asked her to have him call me himself and tell me that I was "fired," but I heard nothing. I telephoned him before the wedding, to assure him that if he needed my help in the days that followed, I would not refuse just because they wanted another minister to officiate. He thanked me and said that he had thought it over and would make a good faith effort to meet with his children and new wife after the wedding. I urged him to do it before the ceremony, but he refused, giving the reason, "I don't want to get upset on the day before my wedding."

Follow-Through

I believe that it is important to follow through to see if the couple do speak directly to parents or others vitally concerned, especially about their tender or angry feelings. In my experience, it is often easier for the couple to tell their parents of their discontents than to simply tell them that they love them and are grateful for everything they have done for them. Good intentions, I have learned, are not enough. I am never completely comfortable in using the moral authority inherent in the clergy role to insist that the task be done. In cases of repeated lies and evasions, I refuse to proceed with the ceremony. I comfort myself by asking if I want to risk my own integrity and self-respect by standing at the altar with a couple about whom statements are made as to their adequacy as adults when they have, in fact, evaded their responsibility. I do not enjoy being disliked, but I do enjoy some new-found self-respect in my conduct as a minister. Moreover, I do not believe any harm is done by the refusal. Couples always seem to find a clergyperson to "do" a wedding.

Using Genetic Information in Premarital Counseling

I have spent some time explaining my approach to premarital counseling before introducing the subjects of genetic information and family health. I am aware of how easily concern about human genetics can be distorted into "eugenics" or unfortunate attempts to "improve" the human species by planned selection of marriage partners. I do not advocate these causes and keep my distance from them. Most premarital counseling has not yet incorporated ways to apply knowledge from human genetics for the couple's benefit in preparing for parenthood. I am a member of the clergy who hopes to improve the chance that the health of children and their parents will be enhanced by incorporating the best insights of the medical, social, and behavioral sciences into pastoral practices, where relevant. Because of the convergence of family and religious process, and because reliable information about the risks of reproduction can be obtained prior to marriage, I believe that all the information that can be reasonably assembled ought to be, in order to provide couples with an opportunity to know themselves and their families better.

Case 9: Discovery of High Genetic Risk After Engagement

The purpose of using genetic information in premarital counseling is to help the couple to be as informed as possible prior to marriage. There should be no coercion or use of clergy authority to influence the couple's reproductive plans, short of being willing to see to it that they know what their options as parents are, in case of significant genetic risk. During the past fourteen years, I have not seen a case in which genetic risk in one or both members of a couple was so high that their marriage plans were affected. However, Aubrey Milunsky reported a case that might have involved a member of the clergy.[5]

Ann was twenty-one years old, engaged to be married soon. Her father had had some kind of disease affecting the brain and nervous system for some years, the name of which had not been told her. The significance of this disease, unfortunately, had also not been communicated to her. Since the disease was in fact Huntington's [disease], serious questions arose when she became informed of all the facts just a few weeks prior to marriage.

Her fiance, of course, had not known either that Ann had a 50 percent chance of actually having Huntington's [disease], or that this disease could slowly appear within a few years after marriage. If his wife indeed had the disease (even though it was not yet apparent) and they had children, then there would be a 50 percent risk that each of their children would develop the same disease. In this case, realization of all the facts led the girl's fiance to break off the relationship and to cancel the marriage. Five years later, sadly, Ann developed Huntington's [disease].

In such a case, if the couple decided to separate due to genetic risks, they would need help to work through the loss of their relationship and its impact on their lives. If the facts of the case were different and Ann and her fiance, having been thoroughly informed, decided to marry and even risk having children, should the clergy counselor go through with the wedding as planned? In my view, genetic risks alone are not a sufficient reason for using the authority of a religious office to try to influence reproductive plans. Religious leaders should not set a precedent of allowing religious institutions to appear to be agents of coercive measures related to human reproduction. My comments here are in the context of a society that has a public policy of freedom with fairness about marriage and reproduction. It would be unfair to Ann and her fiance, if they wanted to be married and take a risk of reproducing, to withhold the ceremony as a price of abstention from increasing risks for their children.

Why would I be willing to withhold my participation in a wedding when the cause is avoidance of honesty in families, and not withhold it when there is a risk that a child may inherit a fatal disease? My answer is this: because there is something the couple can do about remedying the faulty patterns and practices of communication that they learned from parents. There is nothing a couple can do to change their genetic inheritance from their parents. It seems fair to me not to reward a couple for refusing to do something possible that they have already agreed is in their best interests, even if the parents do not listen or change, by giving them the easy way to a "nice wedding" where everyone will smile and nod, but the couple and I will know what has been refused. It seems unfair to me to punish a couple for something they cannot change, the human genotype, even if they intend to proceed with reproduction at great risk. Another version of the same problem would appear if Ann and her fiance knew that their children would be at risk for a disease that could be diagnosed prenatally. There is now no reliable way to diagnose Huntington's disease prenatally. Suppose they told their clergy counselor that, due to moral reasons, they could in no way consider abortion as an option in pregnancy? Would this decision amount to avoidance of responsibility and be a reason for refusing to participate in the wedding? I do not believe so, because the freedom to oppose abortion on moral grounds is, in my view, a sufficient reason to proceed with risks of reproduction, as long as these parents were informed and prepared to accept the consequences. There are clearly two conflicting duties in such a case. Parents have a duty to protect their children, including those not yet born, from harm. Second, there is a duty to protect the freedom of choice and voluntarism that structure the institutions of marriage and family. In this instance, because I believe that safeguarding the freedom that prevails in choices about marriage and reproduction is a higher duty, even if harm might come to children by a lack of coercion of parental freedom, I would not withhold the marriage service. If the parental freedom to use or not to use abortion in reproduction were forbidden or made mandatory, backed up by ecclesiastical sanctions, I believe that the sense that marriage is supposed to make would be corrupted by nonsense coming from, in this example, religious sources. Religious leaders are to safeguard the freedom and fairness on which the assumptions about marriage rest, as long as it is clearly in the best interests of the society to do so. The only scenario in which strong measures about reproduction and marriage customs may be thinkable is when the virtual survival of the society itself is at stake—as, for example, following some biological or atomic disaster, with the extent of destruction of such magnitude as to threaten human evolution itself.

Case 10: Should First Cousins Marry?[6]

The more typical case that the clergy may see in premarital counseling involves people who were of an ethnic group known to be at risk for carrier trait of a genetic disease, or a couple who were cousins and concerned about risks of consanguinity.

A young couple was referred to a genetics clinic by their pastor for genetic counseling. Discussion in a recent premarital interview revealed that Mr. R. and Mrs. R. were first cousins, related through their fathers who were brothers. The couple expressed concern about their background, uncertain as to how this might affect their childbearing. Aside from this worry, the combined families were pleased with the match.

The couple was white and of middle class background; both were professionals. Mr. R. was thirty-two and Mrs. R. twenty-seven; this was a first marriage for each of them. Both were in good health, with no major or prolonged illness or hospitalization for either. Mr. R. was one of three living siblings, one of whom had children, all living and well. Mrs. R. was the oldest of four siblings, none with noteworthy medical problems. Both sets of parents were alive, with the sorts of complaints principally associated with advanced age. There was some, but not an atypical amount, of diabetes mellitus, heart disease, and cancer in the extended kindred, but no unusual early infant deaths or spontaneous abortions or miscarriages, and no mental retardation in any family member. The family originated in Switzerland and had been in this country for several generations.

Counseling of this couple involved essentially the theoretical considerations of consanguinity. It is generally accepted that there is a 3 to 4 percent risk in every pregnancy of a woman having a child with a major birth defect. Epidemiologic studies have shown that, in consanguineous mating, the risk of birth defects is increased by half, or 6 to 8 percent, genetically still considered a low risk. It is also well to bear in mind that, theoretically, a close pooling of genes could well be advantageous to a child, a reassuring notion to be mentioned against the proposed risk figures.

Consanguinity is not an uncommon reason for a couple to seek premarital counseling. Is a marriage between cousins inadvisable? Geneticists tend to disagree on the significance of the added risk of defective offspring. Such factors as the health status of the couple, family background, and perhaps the availability of screening and prenatal diagnosis are important considerations. Finally, however, in the light of the information available, it is the couple that must decide the question.

Historical Perspective on Genetic Information and Religion

Let us consider in a historical perspective the use of genetic information in a religious context. There is a popular idea, probably false, that biblical material in the Mosaic Code (Lev. 18:6–13) concerned with prohibition of incest was *also* related to eugenic concern, namely the knowledge that birth defects are frequent in children born from sexual unions with close relatives. Concern for prevention of birth defects through marriage laws is never directly specified in any biblical text. Incest was treated as a moral offense rather than related to a health concern. The earliest notations about hereditary factors and marriage are from the Talmud, a collection of rabbinic writings that spans over five centuries, beginning in a.d. 400. The Talmud rules that a man may not marry into a family of epileptics or lepers, or a similar disease. David Feldman, a Jewish scholar, states that this may be the "first eugenic edict in any social or religious system."[7] Christian religious laws prohibiting marriage under conditions of consanguinity are ancient, and for the most part they are based upon biblical material. The major religous groups (Roman Catholic, Greek Orthodox, Reformed) differed slightly in terms of the *degree* of relationship within the decendents that was prohibited. The foundations of the reasoning against consanguineous marriages are ethical and social and, in the older authorities, no evidence is given of eugenic concerns.

The most prevalent explanation in the ancient and medieval worlds for the birth of defective children was supernatural.[8] These societies were both repelled and fascinated by so-called "monstrous" births. The earliest societies to keep records (Babylonian, Assyrian, and Egyptian) show that defects were taken to be portents, events that were useful for predicting good or evil events. From North Africa, belief in the supernatural origin and meaning of birth defects spread to Greece, Rome, and Europe. Cicero was a firm believer in divination, and he wrote a long tract on abnormalities as signs of fate or providence. Augury, or the art of divination, played a special role in Roman history. It was from the Latin that the words "portent," "monster," and "prodigy" came into English. The relation of defects to divination continued through the Middle Ages and even into the Protestant Reformation. In 1523, Protestant reformers Martin Luther and Philip Melanchthon published a tract entitled *Der Papstesel*, "The Ass of the Pope." The discovery of a strange "monster" resembling a donkey floating in the Tiber was seen by them as a sign from God meaning the downfall of the Papacy. Actually, someone had tossed the body of a seriously deformed baby, probably with hydrocephalus, into the river.

Another popular theory of birth defects was based on the belief in maternal impressions or frights. Many societies have been found to believe that prenatal mental impressions of the mother can influence the formation of the child, or a sudden shock produce a defect. Being frightened by a rabbit has long been considered the cause of "harelip." Positive impressions could produce healthy children. In Greece, mothers who were expecting were ordered to gaze at statues of Castor and Pollux to make the babies more perfect. In France, it is still the custom for expectant mothers to visit the Louvre.

Birth defects were also associated with theories of demons and witches. Many unfortunate mothers and fathers of newborns with malformations were persecuted or killed for this reason. A hybridity theory developed that accounted for defects due to coupling between humans and animals. In the New Haven Colony in 1642, an innocent one-eyed servant named George Spencer was executed after being found guilty of the birth of a cyclopic (one-eyed) pig with a gigantic snout, clearly an accident of porcine rather than human-animal mating.

Only in relatively modern times (the seventeenth and eighteenth centuries) did an explicit concern with the prevention of birth defects mark Christian writings about marriage between relatives.

These comments were few until the nineteenth century brought more knowledge of comparative anatomy and the environmental causes of malformation. Mendel's laws of heredity, when applied to human genetics, brought a great thrust of further understanding. Even with the addition of new scientific knowledge, ancient superstition about birth defects still haunts modern parents of defective children, as we shall see in the next chapter.

Rationale for Use of Genetic Information in Premarital Counseling

My rationale for the relevance of genetic information in premarital counseling grows out of my earlier discussion of the religious process. "Everybody knows" that parents are supposed to protect children from harm, especially harm that might be prevented by timely action. Additionally, people are supposed to protect themselves from preventable harm. There is also a general social duty to cooperate with physicians and scientists in the prevention of disease.

Although information needed to keep these duties and obligations can be made easily available by noninvasive methods, especially to couples prior to marriage, such is rarely the case. This is due in part to poor education about human genetics and biology. In fact, primary care physicians themselves are only just beginning to learn of the benefits of genetic education and counseling. If there is a general moral obligation or duty to protect the welfare of self and others that is being violated, clergy ought to call attention to the problem. This contradiction ought to provoke awareness, especially among the clergy, whose role includes a responsibility to prepare people for marriage.

Clergy should encourage couples to seek genetic information for two reasons. First, clergy are supposed to be as responsible as anyone else to protect children and parents from the potential harm of accidents of genetics that can be known before birth. Death, as well as great physical and mental suffering, can result from genetic disease. The ethical principle of nonmaleficence is relevant to premarital counseling as well as to the practice of medicine. This principle, generally phrased as *primum non nocere* ("above all, do no harm") has wide acceptance as a central ethical canon of medicine.[9] Clergy, as well as physicians, are supposed to think carefully about the harm that could come to couples directly and indirectly from neglect of emotional and physical responsibilities prior to marriage. By failing to make couples aware of opportunities to learn more about their genetic histories, especially if the resources exist in the local community, clergy can fail in their general and specific duties.

A second reason stems from the principle of veracity that supports a general duty to tell the truth. If one or both members of the couple withhold information that impinges on their health or well-being, could this dishonesty be justified? The following case,[10] composed by educators in genetic counseling, may eventually involve a rabbi's decision about the question.

Case 11: Should I Override Someone's Objections?

A twenty-three-year-old Jewish male is identified, in a large screening program at the university he is attending, as a carrier of a recessive gene for Tay-Sachs disease. During routine couseling, he reveals that he is engaged to a young Jewish woman and is to be married in six months. He also informs the genetic counselor that he has a twenty-year-old sister and a sixteen-year-old brother. After reviewing with the counselor the implications of his carrier status for his future children and his siblings, he steadfastly refuses to inform his fiancée, parents, or siblings of his carrier status, and he tells the counselor that he does not want them informed. What should be the counselor's response?

If the counselor responds by overriding the objections of the groom, in the interests of protecting the health of others, the rabbi who is to be in charge of the ceremony will undoubtedly hear the repercussions. There will be work to do. If the counselor responds by agreeing to remain silent and leave the responsibility to the groom, another scenario could emerge if the rabbi were informed about screening for Tay-Sachs disease and made a practice of raising the issues with couples. What might be the response of the groom in the event the rabbi raised the issue in the context of premarital counseling? In all likelihood, a rabbi sensitive to these matters may be in a position to help the secret be disclosed in a manner that would not lead to punishing feelings by the bride and groom. After all, should we not be more concerned about the real harm that can come to others than the temporary insecurity of revealing a risk that may, in the groom's eyes, threaten his self-esteem? The threat to self-esteem of the discovery that one is a carrier is real. The significance of this threat, however, is not as great as the significance of having the disease or the risk of not knowing that one is a carrier. With proper education and counseling, the significance of the greater threat and the lesser threat can be put into a proper perspective.

The risks to the marriage through neglect of the duty to tell the truth can be significant. If a couple might have known their genetic risks and did not seek seek the knowledge, and if an affected child is born, the chance of them escaping a serious threat to their marriage is very slim. There is a chain of events involved. Lack of attention in premarital counseling to matters of emotional and physical health can be a contributing cause to divorce and separation. Several books now document the serious health consequences, even death, due to loneliness, isolation, and divorce.[11] The work of the clergy can spell the difference between health and illness, life and death.

In my practice of premarital counseling, if a couple were to refuse the requirement to cooperate with me to research their family health histories and consult a physician, I could not conscientiously proceed with helping them to marry. My reason for refusing to continue is that I do not want to take the risk of contributing to preventable harm. Fortunately, no couple to date has refused. On the contrary, couples show a great deal of interest and are grateful for the chance to learn more about their families and themselves.

One way to reduce the impact of resistance to effective premarital counseling is for the clergy to work out policies and standards for the administration of ceremonies and sacraments with the governing body of the congregation. The policies for conduct of funerals, weddings, baptisms, confirmations, and other ceremonies should be carefully defined. Without such policies, clergy could be vulnerable in their own congregations to a troublemaking family that insisted on the wedding taking place in that congregation *or else*.

Clergy who already have or will adopt similar standards for their own conduct are well-advised to make these known to the "search committees" of congregations before taking a new assignment. Clergy who received strong signals that these standards would not be supported by leaders of the congregation would do well to remember that there are other congregations in need of a pastor.

In closing this discussion of premarital counseling, I see the following results of my change in practice:

- The wedding ceremony itself takes on a special significance when the couple, their families, and I have worked hard to clear the air.
- The religious symbolism in the ceremony "speaks" more clearly to the needs that have emerged.
- My wedding sermon (usually five or six minutes) contains reassurances to the couple and the congregation about the personal strength of the couple, based upon real tests, although I do not share the content of the tests. Previously, I never preached at weddings.
- I feel more integrally involved and active in the work of the wedding; as a consequence, I enjoy the ceremony and festivities much more than in the past.
- I have received letters of gratitude from couples, expressing their hope for themselves based upon the lessons they learned about the values that support marriage through working with me.

It does not take many letters of this kind to convince me that the changes have been worthwhile.

4. Counseling the Parents of a Child with a Congenital Malformation

Few events in life result in as much grief and trauma as the birth of a child with a serious congenital malformation. The sorrow and trauma are usually complicated by a sense of guilt in the couple, regardless of whether they were aware of risks. Few events in the work of clergy will be more challenging than the opportunity to participate in the religious process with such parents. This chapter is about counseling parents in this situation and collaborating with the staff of the neonatal intensive care unit (NICU), the special unit in a hospital that provides round-the-clock intensive medical care for high-risk newborns.

The frequency of malformations in the United States is between three and four in every one hundred births. Other reasons why newborns may need intensive care include the following:

- diabetic or drug-addicted mother
- Rh negative mother with rising quantities of Rh antibodies
- delivery by Caesarean section with a variety of complications
- delivery after prolonged labor and fetus has been in distress
- low birthweight infant, either preterm or term
- post-term infants, more than forty-two weeks gestation
- respiratory distress at delivery
- multiple births (e.g., twins, triplets) with potential problems
- infections and jaundice

There are twelve deaths in every one thousand liveborn infants, and permanent handicaps in at least that many at birth. Medical experts in the United States estimate that sixty of every one thousand liveborn infants will need neonatal care.[1] An estimate on the frequency of malformation at birth in the world is "one every thirty seconds."[2]

Learning of the Birth of a Child with Congenital Malformation

In premodern societies, a malformed infant was often abandoned, killed, or ceremonially removed by a religious functionary. Infanticide has been practiced in every part of the world. In 1972, Konner reported on observations of a tribe of African bushpeople, the Zhun-twasi, who bury malformed infants seconds after birth.[3]

In modern society, especially since the nineteenth century, there has been interest in rescuing malformed children from the cruel views and "barbarism" of the past, although our ancestors were not as much motivated by animus towards the malformed infant as by desires to control population and resources, or to balance the sex ratio. With the growth of state and philanthropic interests in treating malformed children wherever possible, better medical and institutional care has enabled many such children to live. Laws in modern nations protect even the most deformed individual. There is now an attitude, broadly shared, that the strong are more a threat to civilization than the weak.

In spite of the growth of a "modern" consciousness about children with birth defects, there is universally a *negative* initial response to the birth of such a child by parents and health professionals. The initial negative reaction, marked by denial and anger, is described by many authorities in the care of parents and newborns. The impact of the affected child creates an "intense crisis," comments an experienced British physician. "Numbness, grief, disgust, waves of helplessness, rage, disbelief are felt; the expected perfect child is lost, and the feared, damaged, deformed child is born. Parents may wish at first to "get rid" of the child, followed by feelings of guilt, self-blame, and intense anxiety."[4]

The initial response of the parents is tempered, however, by different considerations by answers to these questions about the malformation:

- Is it completely correctable or is it noncorrectable?
- Is it visible or nonvisible?
- Does it affect the central nervous system?
- Is it life threatening?
- Will it have an effect on the future development of the child?
- Does it affect the genitalia? The eyes?
- Is it a single or multiple malformation?
- Is it familial?
- Are there other members of the family with a malformation?
- Will there be a need for repeated hospitalizations?
- Will repeated visits to physicians or agencies be needed?[5]

The degree of impairment and the socioreligious situation of the parents condition their response to the child's problem. We know through social research that people believe the most serious defects are "visible," mental handicaps or damage to the head, neck, or face which are not reparable, as opposed to defects which are treatable or out of sight. Also, the experience of serious mental retardation can be devastating if the parents are highly motivated and ambitious for themselves. The child is retarded for everyone to see, and the family's self-concept is jeopardized. Families that are very concerned for their social status are more traumatized by mental retardation.

Protestants are less accepting of mental retardation than Catholics, according to a study of mothers of retarded children.[6] The possibility of an explicit absolution from personal guilt by their religion and the idea that a mother could accept such a child as a test of her religious faith or a "special gift from God" may account for some of the difference. Women have consistently been found more accepting of malformed children than men, a finding that holds true with young girls and boys as well.[7] Since the majority of physicians are males, I expect that there is rejection in the medical profession along the same lines. Since most middle-class families use private physicians to deliver their children, physicians become identified with the family. Those close to the scene of such births know that the physician feels that he or she has failed the family. Physicians' emotions come into play here, probably far more than with lower-class families.

From 1973 to 1975, I served as a consultant and advisor to a neonatal unit in a large metropolitan teaching hospital. I was involved with medical staff, families, clergy, and a counselor employed by the hospital to work with the parents of seriously ill infants. I learned firsthand about the swirling, confusing emotions that well up in everyone concerned with the infant's welfare, and in myself.

In the cases in which I was involved, I noted that the first reaction to the news was one of *numbness*, followed by withdrawal. The numbness was then replaced by a tendency to *deny* the seriousness of the defect. The parent's attitude was, "the physicians are mistaken." A second or third opinion was often requested. In the past, the mother was shielded at first by grogginess from anesthesia, but in modern hospitals both mother and father are alert at time of birth. They hear as much as the medical staff about the infant's condition. But they do not believe what they hear. They repeat to themselves over and over, "It can't be true." Physicians and nurses are accustomed to this denial and patiently keep pressing the parents to accept the truth. Sometimes time is short, due to the severity of the defect, and decisions need to be made about treatment. As the truth sinks in, the parents become very angry. They are angry at themselves, at the child, and (even though they may be agnostic) angry at God or the fate that brought them to this pass. They are angry with staff physicians and nurses. They are angry at the false reassurance given by unwitting physicians during pregnancy. Nancy Irvin and colleagues report an interview with a woman whose child had Down syndrome. She was one in a series of mothers with affected children whom they studied to find creative ways to respond to this crisis. Irvin wrote that almost every mother so interviewed talked about disturbing dreams that the fetus she was carrying was malformed. They remember being afraid that the dream was literal. The woman, whose name was changed in the report, mentioned her experience in bringing up the subject of her fear with her obstetrician:

Mrs. Cook: But I did mention it to Dr. L., my obstetrician, three or four months before Walter was born, and he just said, "Oh no, no way, no way could this ever be," and he just reassured me. Later I again approached him on it and he comforted me, "No way, no way."[8]

We do not know for sure what Dr. L. said to her, but she remembers being falsely reassured. Apparently, the anxiety that marks the religious process in childbirth begins for many women long before delivery. The experience of false reassurance shows the need for realistic facing of risks, followed by reassurance that, given the worst possibility, physicians do have ways to help.

If the infant's disease is treatable or not severe enough to call into question the prolongation of life, the hospital staff will "re-present" the infant to the parents. The new, damaged child, is presented as a substitute for the lost, ideal child. If the parents can reorganize their loyalties to the lost child, and respond with love for the new child, there is a good chance they can recover from the crisis. But it can take many months for some parents to recover their balance as human beings, and for the injury to their self-esteem and confidence in the goodness of life to be repaired. Not the least problem in this period is the sincere wish by the parents for the child's death.

The goal of the work of physicians, nurses, and psychological counselors during this period is to help the suffering parents develop new attachments to the malformed infant. The relevance of creative participation in the religious process that coincides with this medical and therapeutic aid should be plain. The stakes are high, and they include the well-being of the child as well as of the parents. As Bruno Bettelheim wrote:

Children can learn to live with a disability. But they cannot live without the conviction that their parents find them utterly loveable. . . . If the parents, knowing about his [the child's] defect, love him now, he can believe that others will love him in the future. With this conviction, he can live well today and have faith about the years to come.[9]

The religious process can issue in a type of love that was kindled in the fires of suffering, purged of all false hope, reborn on the other side of despair, and premised on a source of help outside the self. Religious traditions have called this type of love *agape*, from the Greek word that differentiates this type of love from *philia*, what friends feel for one another. *Agape* is the Greek word in the Bible that translates the Hebrew word *aheb*. The meaning of the word is "the mercifulness of God."

The Religious Process in the Crisis Following the Birth of a Child with Congenital Malformations

Physicians such as Marshall Klaus and John Kennell, who pioneered creative ways of working with parents in this crisis, charted the emotional experience of parents in terms that appear in Figure 12. This outline not only highlights the salient features of the experience of being with parents and others in the NICU, it also

Fig. 12. Hypothetical model of the sequence of normal parental reactions to the birth of a child with congenital malformations

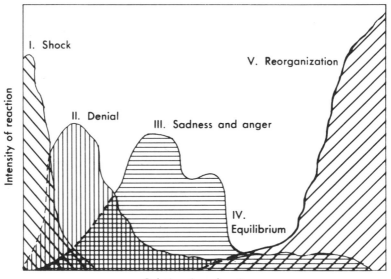

SOURCE: D. Drotar, et al., *Pediatrics* 56, no. 5 (Nov. 1975), pp. 710–717. Copyright © American Academy of Pediatrics 1975.

resembles, I believe, the general parabolic shape of the religious process wherever it appears in human life.

The "shock" permeates and numbs not only their emotions but, in my experience, strikes a blow at the heart of their standing in the human community. The self-esteem of the parents is deeply injured. What greater blow is there than to give oneself to the long preparation for bearing a child, imagining what that child will be like, allowing the new trust and confidence in one's adequacy to be a parent to emerge, and *then* have those hopes dashed? The blow is not only personal, but ontological. The parents feel assaulted and injured by a cosmic force or God. The guilt that they suffer is not only personal but a feeling that they have offended their obligation to the universe to be adequate parents. "Why did this happen to me?" is a question that reveals the turbulent feelings that provoke the religious process.

Some reflection on the developments of pregnancy will lay the groundwork for considering the religious significance of this particular crisis. The process of pregnancy involves stages in which both parents undergo profound changes to prepare them for acceptance of their parental roles. Energy and commitment must be released from other objects and people so that they can care adequately for the child. They imagine what the child will be like, and how they will be as parents. Using an analogy from the Christian calendar, this Advent period is filled with expectations that prepare them for the "coming."

The profundity of parents' and their families' grief when a child is born with a serious malformation reflects the symbolic impact of a ruined natality event. Hannah Arendt eloquently argued that two of the basic conditions of human life, action and work, are deeply rooted in the birth events of mankind. Natality events, in every culture, are the focus for hope that the inexorable laws of mortality and the cycle of the biological process are not the final comments on the meaning of human existence.

The miracle that saves the world, the realm of human affairs, from its normal, "natural" ruin is ultimately the fact of natality, in which the faculty of action is ontologically rooted. It is, in other words, the birth of new men and the new beginning, the action they are capable of by virtue of being born. Only the full experience of this capacity can bestow upon human affairs faith and hope. . . .[10]

Robert Jay Lifton's studies of "symbolic immortality" include childbirth as one mode of immortality, in which "experiential transcendence" occurs. People thereby transcend the ordinary limits of time and daily life.[11] The biological and cultural process of pregnancy prepares the parents, especially the mother, for the appearance of a unique individual. It seems that all of the cultural and biological systems of humans work together to prepare for the child who appears with the force of a miracle, or at least as the center of an event that has the capacity to elevate parents and their helpers beyond the cloying, downward pull of everyday.

What happens when the child presents itself with a serious malformation from which no real recovery is likely? The initial, universally negative reaction to the child unites everyone in confrontation with the terror of death even in the sublime moment of birth. At the initial response, nothing is wanted other than that the reminder of death and finitude be gone. It is in the second response, when the different authority and reference groups to which all respond come into play, that the moral debate begins. What should we do for the child? After the initial shock has passed, we know that decisions must be made within the possibilities that training, ethics, and resources make available. The profound ambivalence towards the malformed newborn can be understood as a struggle within the tension of a first emotional response to be rid of the child and the injury to the ideal arrangements that have been made, and a second, more socialized response to behave in a way that transforms the "nonsense" of wanting the child dead. It is honest to admit the wish to be rid of the child, but we ought not to act on the wish. We can also say, without fear of contradiction, that doing so would not rid us of the terror of death.

I once visited a mother following the birth of a second child with a serious genetic disorder. As she wept and vented her sense of failure as a mother, she cried, "Why does God do such terrible things to children! After the first one was born, I prayed to God not to let this happen again, and just look at what happened!" As she talked on, she commented, "You spend all your life looking at pictures of pretty babies and their mothers and growing up thinking that will be you. It is pretty gruesome when you are the one who is different."[12]

You are the one who is different. It does not make sense, when you have put your trust in the arrangements by which "everyone knows" what is supposed to happen when you get pregnant. Americans tend to expect the perfect baby. We may be aware of birth defects, but they will happen to someone else's baby.

There are few human losses that can do more injury to the human ability to respond than the birth of a malformed child. In my experience, it is surpassed only by the sudden death of an apparently normal infant, or the suicide of a son or daughter. Guilt following these calamaties is more paralyzing because the parents believe themselves culpable. Now that techniques help to to diagnose more disorders in the fetus, parents will feel culpable for having not used the techniques, especially if something might have been done during pregnancy to help the future child, or to help themselves consider other options, including abortion, earlier in pregnancy.

The Clergy Role in Counseling Parents of an Infant with Congenital Malformation

Clergy are needed in this situation because it is a religious, as well as emotional and ethical, crisis. The role of the clergy is to be faithful companions who encourage participation in the religious process and model this participation by their own decisions and behavior while helping others. Above all, the clergy need not talk *about* the religious process. The proper concern should be to recognize what is going on, leading and participating at the same time.

Actually, the religious process begins long before the climax of birth, in the events and changes of pregnancy. Pregnancy changes a woman's previous standing in the community. She needs help and cooperation from others that exceed the normal routine of everyday life. Her husband needs help to accept the change in her and its implications for him. The early stirrings of anxiety and bad dreams about malformations need to be faced, not erased superficially by false reassurance. The shock of jealousy in the husband, mixed with pride, also needs to be faced.

I have seen clergy wait with fathers outside the delivery room to receive word about the health of mother and child. I was impressed with the difference their companionship can make. The advantage of being present is that a call is not needed in case of trouble. Clergy also have the advantage of seeing the events unfold firsthand rather than be told later by someone else, and perhaps be misinformed about the trouble.

An alternative to waiting with the father, now that fathers participate in the delivery in many cases, is to arrange to be called by a nurse on duty. Clergy can lay the groundwork for being an effective companion to the staff as well as to parents in the Ob-Gyn area of a hospital or the NICU. Early in their assignment to a new town or city, and as part of making themselves known to hospital staff and authorities, the clergy can visit the newborn nursery and the NICU. Clergy should get acquainted and acknowledge that they expect to work closely with the staff on behalf of the parents in the congregation in the events of childbirth. Clergy should ask if they can be included on rounds at a convenient time in the future, in order to meet physicians and nurses together, see the unit, and get an impression of the ambience in which decisions are made. Many clergy feel like strangers in a hospital, especially with the staff. There is something the clergy can do to prevent this feeling and ensure that when there is trouble, they can begin working on the other side of the role of newcomer. After all, medical staffs have good reason to be wary of clergy, or anyone else for that matter, who are perfect strangers to them.

The first responsibility of the clergyperson is to be as honest *with self* as possible about the feelings that are provoked by the event. Some clergy imitate physicians or psychiatrists in such situations, probing for the feelings of others and asking them to expose their feelings. Why go down this path? There is also the danger of being seduced by the medical details. Clergy couselors may take the lead in expressing the shock, pain, and anger that is real, especially if they are close to the couple by virtue of companionship in the past. Then, if the clergy want to be of help, they must ask the couple if they want their help, not only in the beginning, but throughout the various parts of the crisis.

If the couple says no, which is unlikely, the probabilities are (1) the shock and numbness are talking; (2) they are angry at the cler-gyperson, especially if all of that person's children are healthy; or (3) they do not know what kind of help the clergy has to offer. They also may guard their own autonomy and be wary of any threat to their independence. One must always be prepared to let go and not help.

If the couple say yes, the likelihood is that the dam holding their feelings will break along with saying yes. As they talk, the tasks are (1) to be sure they help one another face the feelings, and (2) that feelings about others not present (e.g., physicians, nurses, grand-parents, the child, God) are eventually communicated directly.

One counselor in an NICU helped couples face their feelings about the child by placing a pillow in the lap of the mother and asking her to imagine it to be the child. She was encouraged to say whatever came to mind. Often this helped to release the wish that the baby would die. I myself, when the mother or husband expressed anger at God, have urged them to express it themselves in prayer, if they believed that God hears prayers, or in any other way that made sense to them.

If the NICU has a counselor or liaison psychiatrist whose respon-sibilities include helping parents with their injured feelings, the clergy counselor should see to it that he or she is involved in a joint meeting with the parents. It may also happen that the other profes-sional will ask the clergyperson to be involved. If the unit lacks this resource person, the clergy are well-advised to involve a nurse or physician in the process of facing feelings, because anger that remains inside, unexpressed to medical staff of the NICU, can go "underground" and emerge later to sabotage the decisionmaking about treatment or nontreatment for the most seriously ill infants.

Another important reason to help self and parents face the pain and anger behind the numbness is that they cannot "hear" very well the information physicians must tell them about the child's condi-tion until their responses to their own injuries begin to flow again. Some physicians can be insensitive to the need to wait, before de-scribing the details of the problem, until the parents' ability to re-spond to more information has been tested. When the clergy counselor actually sees the parents' eyes glaze and the physician keeps talking past them, nothing will be hurt by saying something like, "I don't know about you, but I don't understand it and I need to talk about why."

Facing painful feelings is not a once and for all experience. It needs to be done in each new context and stage in the crisis. The next problem will involve decisions to treat the infant, or to begin a trial of treatment to see if the infant responds. The prevailing ethic in NICUs in the United States is to give the high-risk infant the benefit of any doubt about starting treatment or a trial treatment. Neonatologists, in my experience, do not "trade off" the infant's chance for treatment for considerations about money, societal burdens, or even the parents' adequacy to care for the infant. These issues are real, and they have some weight in the total scheme of things, but the working standard in the NICU is to "try." Medically, this standard makes sense, because the infant's ability to respond needs to be tested. If the response is poor, it may follow that another path needs to be chosen, namely, a succession of decisions to support the infant technologically until the evidence is clear that nothing else ought to be done except prepare for the infant's death, or to refer the infant to another facility for long-term care.

However, what makes medical sense to neonatologists may be nonsense to parents whose hopes have been dashed. The clergy counselor may have the opportunity to be involved in the decision about therapy, as a companion to the parents and the staff, if such help is sought. The following case report from my records illustrates the dynamics of the treatment decision and how I understood my role.

Case Report: Baby Boy with Down Syndrome and Duodenal Stenosis

I received a call from Ms. A., a counselor in a neonatology unit of a local hospital. Her role was to work with the emotional aspects of decisionmaking about the treatment of newborns with serious disease and handicaps. She and I had been associated in several cases with parents and physicians.

She asked me if I would be a consultant on ethics to a meeting of the staff about their disagreements on what to do about a baby boy born with Down syndrome and duodenal stenosis. X-ray showed a partial closure of the esophagus. The infant was being fed by mouth, and retained some and vomited some. The question was whether to operate on the stenosis. The parents were now opposed to the surgery, and the staff was divided. The physician in charge of the unit, Dr. L., had been newly appointed. He had done his training and residency in that hospital. This was his first major case of this type since being appointed head of the unit. Dr. L. had encouraged Ms. A. to call me. I said that I would be a consultant at the meeting. Could I meet the parents and understand their views? She assured me that I could. The parents, Mr. and Mrs. T., were both at the hospital with the baby. I could come anytime.

The counselor told me that the parents had changed their minds about treatment. This was their first child and Down syndrome was a great shock to them. At first, they thought that they must have the operation, and that they had no legal or moral choice in the matter. They met with a pediatric surgeon who pointed out that they did have an option to oppose the surgery. This request had caused a serious ethical controversy among the staff.

I vividly recall walking into the NICU of the hospital. Mr. and Mrs. T. stood by the crib of their baby. They looked limp and forlorn. Mr. T. especially looked defeated. I introduced myself and said that Ms. A. had called me, with Dr. L.'s agreement, and asked me to be a consultant for a staff meeting later to discuss the alternatives in the treatment of their baby. I wanted to talk with them both and get their views. Mr. T. began immediately to describe the baby's medical problems. I interrupted and suggested that we go into another room to talk.

We went into a sitting room outside the nursery. Mrs. T.'s eyes and face were red from crying. When we sat down, she began to cry again. "I'm sorry," she said, "I can't stop crying." "What's there to be sorry for about crying?" I answered. I continued, "I'm sad, too, because I have gotten myself into a situation here where I realize that you were not asked if you wanted a consultant beyond the help that you have. I have agreed to work with the doctors, but I should have asked Ms. A. to ask you if you wanted my help." I apologized to them both for neglecting their choice in the matter. They accepted the apology and said that they were willing to go over their thinking with me.

Mrs. T. began, saying, "The first thing I want to say is that I am about to scream at the nasty way I am being treated by some of the nurses and doctors in the nursery. When I go in to look at the baby,

I can feel them looking at me with hatred. They know that my husband and I have seriously questioned the value of an operation and they are trying to make me feel guilty." Mr. T. was quiet, observing his wife carefully. I asked him, "What is your advice to your wife about that?" He looked surprised, stunned. "What do you mean?" he asked. "You know Mrs. T. better than I do," I replied. "How would you help her with her problem? It must be tough to have taken a controversial position and then be treated with contempt." He thought and then suggested, "I suppose you could say to them, I would like it better if you went ahead and said out loud what you think." "What do you think about that?" I asked Mrs. T. She thought that it was good advice.

They then covered the same ground Ms. A. had covered earlier. After their discussion with the surgeon, they realized that what they really wanted "for the baby's sake" was no treatment. They did not want the baby "to suffer." Mr. T. also spoke of a "right to health" that the infant could never enjoy. I said that it was certainly true that some thinkers and writers had argued that to allow such infants to die was a more merciful alternative to a life of mental retardation. But, I could tell them with confidence that these thinkers and writers were definitely in the minority of prevailing ethical views. I said that the surgeon was entitled to his interpretation of the issue, but that they, at least, ought to clarify their own ethical position as sharply as possible. "I am here to get your views so I can do the best job in the staff meeting, so I would appreciate it if you told me what *you* want and why you want it."

"But that's what we've been doing," rejoined Mr. T. "No, you haven't," I answered. "You have been telling me in effect what you think your baby would want if he could speak for himself, which is impossible. As long as you use the infant as a person to speak through, I can't understand you. Try to speak for yourselves, without using the baby as a substitute for the word 'I.' "

There was a long silence. Both Mr. and Mrs. T. looked at the floor. Nothing came forth. "May I ask you some questions about yourselves and your families?" I asked. "You have a counselor, Ms. A. She has asked me to help her and the staff. I need to understand you better in order to be of help." Each said that it would be all right. Neither had any history of genetic disease in the immediate family background. Each had wanted the baby and planned for the conception. Then I asked, "What are you aware of right now? Don't worry about making sense." Mrs. T., without any hesitation, said angrily, "No one in his family has even been here to see me or the baby. That is what I am aware of." Mr. T. was smiling. "I don't see why you are smiling," I said. "What she described is not very pretty."

Mr. T. looked at me in a hurt and puzzled way. I asked Mrs. T., "Are you proud of him for the way he is acting about his family?" She looked down and almost whispered, "No, I'm not." "Tell him, not me," I asked her. She said, "I'm not proud of you. My mother can't be here with me. She is sick in another city. I have not seen one member of your family." She began to cry.

Mr. T. said, "It's my mother. She doesn't understand. She thinks there is a genetic problem here that she had something to do with. I know that she doesn't want the baby to live." I asked him how he knew it, and he answered that he had talked to his mother by telephone. "What happened between you on the telephone?" I asked. Mr. T. said, "She got very upset when I told her what was wrong with the baby, and she blamed herself. She thinks that there was something wrong with her or something she did that made this happen. She said that it would be better if the baby died. She started crying and then hung up." Even at this point, Mr. T. had a smile on his face as he talked. I asked him, "Do you know that you are smiling?" "No," he answered. "Smiling is very confusing to me," I said, "because what you are telling me is sad." I asked if he had called his mother to say that he and Mrs. T. needed her and that they want her to come to learn about the real reasons the baby is sick. "No," Mr. T. answered. "I figured, why upset her even more?"

I told the couple at this point that although they had not asked for my help as a counselor, I did have a recommendation to make, if they were interested. They said that they were. I said to Mr. T., "You need to act now to have your mother and members of your family come to the hospital, and you need to meet with Ms. A. and Dr. L.. Go over the medical facts. Get this business with your mother's guilt out in the open."

He stood up and walked to the window. "You don't understand," he said. "My mother is a very difficult person. She has acted this way for years." I said to him, "I came to you to ask your views about your baby. What you have given me so far are what *others* have said, or what you think the baby would want. You let the baby do your talking for you. I am concerned that you might think nothing at all except what you pick up from other people as signals. I think you need to take some action on a problem that you can do something about, like your mother's hostile treatment of you and your wife. Do something about that and then pay attention to the problem of the baby again. You might then be more able to know your own mind. You are not able now to speak for yourselves, not only because you are hurt and confused, but because you are paralyzed. You can't even get up the energy to solve this little problem of your mother's reaction. How are you going to make the bigger decision about the baby's life?" I stopped and waited.

Mr. T. was silent, but his smiles disappeared. He looked angry and resentful. I turned to his wife, "Do you understand, Mrs. T.? I am saying that I do not think you two can speak clearly about what you want until you do something first about the pain and chaos you feel. His family is only part of it. Do you understand me?" She spoke up crisply, "I certainly do." I asked, "Do you want your husband to take charge and get his family over here?" She said, "I certainly do." "Then tell him directly," I said. She turned to him and said, "Please help me and yourself. I can't take any more of this kind of thing!" He stood up and said that he would get on the telephone. I left and went to Dr. L.'s office.

I found Dr. L. in a very agitated state. He had heard a rumor that an organization for parents of Down syndrome children had inquired about the case. Officials in the hospital had been alerted. Wheels were in motion that could take the case out of his hands. There was a hospital ethics committee that could be called in to make a decision, if need be. "We will see," I said. "In the meantime, do you want to have the staff meeting?" He was affirmative. "Well, then, I must know what you think about this case. What do you want?" Dr. L. said, "I want to be fair. I want to respect their views, they are entitled to them. My view is that if it were my baby, I would operate. I don't think this is severe enough to warrant withholding surgery." I asked him if he had told the parents what he had told me. He had. Dr. L. said that the conflict on the staff was intense and deep. He wanted me to draw people out and to help the group examine the best arguments on both sides of the issue. Before we went into the staff meeting, I asked Dr. L. if he were interested in my impressions of the way he was acting. He said, "I think so." I said, "You strike me as a person who is bending over backwards to be fair. You have certain feelings about the option of nontreatment that you are not being open about. You need to say more about what is on your mind."

Approximately twenty people had gathered for the meeting. There were physicians, nurses, hospital officials, and social workers who had been invited by Ms. A. and Dr. L. to discuss the case. All were involved in the neonatal unit in some way. Dr. L. introduced me as a consultant in bioethics whom he had asked to assist with the meeting. I opened the meeting briefly with a word of praise for Dr. L. and Ms. A. in arranging a meeting to be sure that everyone was heard. I said that there was only one rule and that was to say "what was on your mind and your feelings." One by one, everyone spoke. Every aspect of the case was discussed in the next two hours. The ethical, legal, and medical facts were exhaustively covered.

Some nurses were bitter that they were watching parents "abandon" the baby. Other nurses were sympathetic to the parents. The ethical issue boiled down to one basic judgment: was mental retardation itself a sufficient condition to warrant nontreatment? On that the group divided, but the majority were for treatment. Those in the minority believed that "quality of life" standards could legitimately be used to justify letting the baby die. Those who opposed that step challenged the proponents as to whether anyone would be willing to give the baby a lethal dose of morphine or some other substance. No one picked up the challenge.

The hospital administrator reminded the group that the law was very strict on nontreatment of infants. Manslaughter and child abuse were at issue. He thought that the hospital ethics committee should meet about it. During all of this period, Dr. L. had not really spoken his mind. He was listening to the others, asking a question here and there, but essentially waiting for both sides to have their say. The meeting became heated at one point. One young physician accused the others of entertaining "cold-blooded murder." I reminded him that he did have the option of taking himself off the case, if he felt that strongly about the issue. He was silent for a moment, thinking about the matter, and then stated that he could no longer conscientiously serve on the case, if the nontreatment option were seriously considered as a viable alternative. Dr. L. finally spoke, saying that he preferred the option of an operation, but he still wanted to respect the parents' views. The meeting wound down. I stated that very good and moral people differed on cases of this kind. I tested them further by describing two policy options. One would have them treat all Down syndrome cases, without exception. The second made exceptions for nontreatment, including parental desires for nontreatment when there were no other deficit except mental retardation. They did not want to adopt any policy, but take decisions on a case-by-case basis.

People in the room shifted uneasily. I could tell that there was a need for a decision to be made by the leader, Dr. L. He remained quiet. I spoke again, addressing him by name, with the question, "What are you going to do?" Dr. L. said, "I am going to watch the baby carefully for the time being. I am going to feed the baby by mouth. There is a small amount of food getting through on account of some evidence of bowel movement. Meanwhile, we continue to talk about the options." The meeting ended.

I felt very uneasy and guilty at the end of the meeting. I knew that there was more I wanted and needed to say. I did not think that the parents' desires should be given with as much moral weight as Dr. L. had assigned to them, but I had gotten myself into a situation, along with Dr. L., of trying to be "fair" to the parents. I feared that Dr. L. would either run into legal trouble or have the case taken out of his hands by a superior who would use the reason that he was inexperienced at this "dicey" kind of decisionmaking.

I returned to the hospital two days later to find that Mr. and Mrs. T were more concerned that the baby was suffering through collective inaction. Dr. L. assured them that such was not the case. The baby was neither gaining nor losing weight. Dr. L. explained to me that waiting a bit longer would not hurt the infant. He hoped that nothing more serious would develop. Meanwhile, the hospital ethics committee had met with Dr. L. and had not required him to bring the matter to a quick decision. He commented that the committee deliberated more on its proper functions than on the case.

Mr. T. had insisted that his mother and close relatives come to the hospital to see the child and his wife, which they had done. Mr. T., his mother, and Mrs. T. consulted a geneticist who helped correct the grandmother's misplaced guilt.

One week passed. Mr. and Mrs. T. could no longer bear the risk of waiting longer and requested surgery. Surgery was uneventful and the baby recovered sufficiently to be taken home. I had no further contact with Mr. and Mrs. T. after my second visit. I had more contact with Dr. L. and Ms. A. that proved to be very educational to us. Dr. L. and I are of the same mind at this date, that we both acted in the interests of being "fair," but we now believe that a more aggressive approach to treatment should have been taken earlier. Dr. L. recalls the "great sense of relief" that came over him and his coworkers when a decision was made to operate. The one regret I have is not including the parents in the staff meeting. It now seems obvious, but I did not think of it then.

My own moral position with respect to this particular medical condition was greatly clarified by this case. Mental retardation associated with Down syndrome is not profound enough in itself (and uncomplicated by any other physical problems) to warrant nontreatment. The child's life need not be overwhelmed by the disease, especially if the child has good care in a concerned family. Parents should be persuaded to accept this particular damaged child as an acceptable substitute for their lost, ideal child. In the event of their refusal to consent to the operation, medical authorities could seek legal remedies and persuade the parents to forego their parental responsibilities. Others are willing to adopt retarded children and substitute for the lost parents. There are many conditions more serious than Down syndrome, however, that can warrant decisions not to bring treatment or discontinue a trial of treatment.

When parents take home a child who has a major malformation, they, other children, and the extended family will need to reach deeply for resources to cope with the many problems and concerns that arise. The additional help of members in a congregation who can assist in the care or even replace the parents for a few hours' respite will be greatly welcomed.

Counseling in Decisions to Allow to Die

Our society places the responsibility to make the "lead" decision about discontinuing treatment or not beginning treatment upon physicians. In the medical process, the physician is supposed to be the therapeutic leader and usually is the first to initiate discussion of the lack of therapeutic alternatives when a trial of treatment has failed. Because so many therapeutic options are available in the NICU, neonatologists and pediatricians are activist in their approach to the high-risk infant. In the present arrangements of medicine, activism can be justified. The moral policy that structures expectations in the NICU is "give the baby the benefit of the doubt" until there is medical evidence that "trying" no longer makes sense.

I have observed that two types of problems intrude in these arrangements. The first is competition for the attending physician's leadership in the decisionmaking. For reasons that probably have to do with poor morale and a lack of direct communication in the NICU staff, disagreement with physicians' decisions, especially by nurses, can be readily picked up by the parents and their companions. Mr. and Mrs. T. were both aware of these disagreements. I have seen nurses in an NICU talk to parents about other alternatives without having consulted the physician about their intention to speak to the parents. If the clergy counselor sees this kind of "end-run" by a member of the staff, steps should be taken to correct the problem. First of all, the nurse should be made aware of the trouble he or she is making.

Sometimes physicians encourage the tendency in others to "take over" by not allowing enough time for discussion of the case, or by not inviting nurses as well as physicians to challenge a position. If a clergy counselor is associated with a NICU for any length of time, there will be many opportunities to give the medical head of the unit the benefit of such observations. It is wise to begin this discussion by asking the physician if he or she is interested in one's observations, and if so, to give them concisely without recommendations unless requested.

A second kind of problem makes a caricature of the arrangements for the informed consent of parents to treatment and nontreatment

decisions for the infant. I have seen more than one physician pro-
crastinate about keeping parents abreast of their infant's clinical
situation. Perhaps the physician will do a good job of consulting
colleagues and nurses, but be uncomfortable with parents, especially those who are very angry and punishing about their suffering.
The physician can avoid informing such parents, but avoidance will
be to their detriment. I was made aware of a case in which physicians were themselves actively considering discontinuing treatment
of a heavily brain-damaged infant. The parents were not aware of
the facts of the matter, and it was clear that they were going to be
shocked to hear how badly the child had deteriorated. When I
reminded the physicians of the danger they were in, they fell back
on their observations of "marital problems of this couple." I coun-
tered immediately by saying that they themselves were contributing
to marital problems by withholding important information from the
couple. They corrected the deficiency straight away.

As the therapeutic options narrow and exhaust themselves, it
becomes desirable to stop trying and accept the better way of preparing for the eventual death of the infant. Sometimes the infant's
death follows the simple act of disconnecting a respirator. In most
cases, however, many painful choices lie ahead about what to withhold, whether the alternatives cause the infant pain, and how the
infant is to be fed. There are so many approaches to pain and feeding the infant that it is considered unethical to deprive infants of
medication and at least low level intravenous feeding, even while
more life-prolonging alternatives are being discontinued. Is this ethically dishonest and disingenuous? Would it not be more merciful
to withhold absolutely everything or even to hasten the death by
injecting a lethal dose?

This is not the place to make a full-scale ethical argument against
active euthanasia.[13] Simply, there are two reasons why the good that
might be done to end quickly the suffering of the child is out-
weighed by the harm that would be done by pediatric euthanasia.
The first is an ethical reason that requires no religious backing for
its support.[14] The second is a theological reason that can accompany
the ethical argument against euthanasia.

The only circumstances in which infanticide might imaginably be
justified would be those that resemble the primitive, deprived con-

ditions of the bushpeople who practice it today. If a group of survivors on a remote island with little food included two or more expectant mothers, and several surviving children of mothers who had drowned, and if one mother gave birth to a very malformed or sickly infant, the conditions might present themselves for a decision to end quickly the life of the newborn. Others would starve if no action were taken. But in the context of the modern hospital, even with the most prolonged life of a newborn, it would clearly be unethical for physicians to harm a child by killing. Besides the additional harm and pain caused to the victim by killing, the experience of killing is brutalizing for all involved. Physicians are not educated ethically to kill. Additionally, killing would cause added suffering and guilt for the parents, who deserve to feel that "everything reasonable" that could be done was done. It is unthinkable that public attitudes would encourage any pediatric euthanasia or accept any act of active euthanasia, even if parents begged for it in the name of mercy, simply because the harm that would be done to many others so far outweighs the temporary relief from suffering that might be gained for parents and physicians, or the ending of the child's suffering.

The strongest theological argument against active euthanasia, in my view, is that killing a human being is a denial of the help that God gives, even in the direst conditions in which euthanasia could be ethically justified, to withstand the desire to kill in the name of mercy and simply thank God for every moment of the life of a human being. Human survival is rooted more in the long run in trust in a Creator of life than on the ethical powers of humans to reason about the conditions under which survival can be justified. The "courage to be" does not finally arise from debatable ethical beliefs, but from trust in an indestructible source of mercy (agape) that is incompatible with a practice of killing human beings who are suffering.

If a Child Dies

If the child is to die in the hospital, clergy counselors can take the initiative in helping the couple, in cooperation with the medical staff, prepare for its death and the aftermath. Under normal condi-

tions in the NICU, death is "failure" and embarrasses the physicians and nurses. Success is standing at the door with the recovered
infant and turning him or her over to the radiant parents to take
home. Because the notion of successfully participating in the dying,
death, and mourning of an infant is exceptional in many (but not
all) medical circles, physicians and nurses are uncomfortable at first
but eventually happy for any help they receive from clergy, whose
task it is to represent the strength that holds human confidence
together when nothing else can.

By the time an infant or young child begins to die, even one with
a major malformation, he or she is felt to be a member of the
family. Bonds of affection have formed that require separation and
resolution if the family is to move ahead with hope. Experienced
clergy know that there are actually many interdependent parts in
the religious process that emerge in dying, burial, and mourning.
Figure 13 is a description of the events and stages in the religious
process in mourning. Mourning often begins with the realization
that "nothing more can be done" to prevent the infant's death.
Another point from which to date the emergence of mourning is
with the birth of the malformed child, but this can vary depending
on the type of impairment.

The tasks of the clergy companion will be varied and difficult

Fig. 13. The religious process in mourning

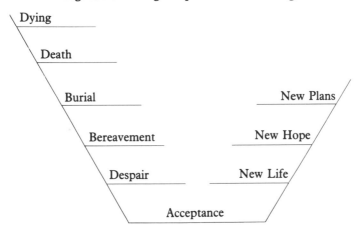

during the entire period, but the tasks are possible because the religious process itself provides a structure for the work. The first problem is usually denial of the dying. It helps greatly to overcome denial if couples have physical contact or at least visual contact with the dying infant. Some physicians may show fear or loathing about the prospect of parents touching the infant before death. Kennell did a study in 1970 of the emotional well-being of mothers after touching the baby before death.[15] He reported no pathological consequences, except that one mother who failed to touch an infant who had previously died had a pathological reaction when a second infant died.

The family should have been gathered together prior to the decision not to continue any trial of therapy, so that they will feel consulted and there will be no secrets about what is to happen. Parents can use discretion about which children to involve directly in this time, but in my experience, no harm comes to children whose parents want them to know what they know. Raymond Duff and his colleagues in the NICU at Yale–New Haven Hospital in New Haven, Connecticut, often assemble the family as a group, if possible, with the damaged infant, so that everyone hears the same thing.[16]

Another opportunity to gather the family is when a critically ill, dying infant is baptized. If death is imminent, it is better that the family remain together until the infant dies, because the second problem in the process is accepting the reality of the infant's death. Practices in a hospital do not lend themselves to success in acceptance of the reality of death. Klaus and Kennell write about these practices and their effects on one mother:

> When a newborn dies in the hospital, all evidence of his existence is usually removed with amazing rapidity, and nothing is left to confirm the reality of his death. "Everything just happened so fast . . . my mind kept going around in circles. I didn't really understand," said one mother. "Just last Sunday I was thinking about her, thinking that my husband and I were the only ones who saw her—its like there is no proof there ever was a baby. We were the only ones who ever saw her and it was just for a couple of days. When a baby dies that small, there's no funeral, no masses. It seems like sort of a shame that there isn't something more. . . . I felt I was on an island by myself . . . lost.[17]

The major function of burial is to "confirm the reality of . . . death" by helping the survivors to say goodbye with their hearts as well as their minds to the one who has died. In my own practice at funerals and burials in the past fourteen years, I have found it invaluable for the extended family to meet on the night before the ritual. We talk about the person who died, as much as those there desire. People weep and sigh. They hold and comfort one another. I encourage the oldest sons and daughters to take the initiative to help family members with grudges or old hurts to talk about the problem and give forgiveness a chance. Expressions of guilt can be directly answered. I also ask a person close to the one who died to say something for the family at the service. By preparing for the service and expressing grief well before it, the symbolic help that the service has to offer is much clearer and "rings true." There should be funeral and burial rites for infants who die, in my view, because the mourning that normal adults and children do for them is very similar to mourning for relatives who live much longer. Observers of parents in this situation comment that a four- to six-month mourning period is normal. Kennell noted that symptoms were "sadness, loss of appetite, insomnia, preoccupation with thoughts of the infant, irritability, and loss of normal behavior patterns."[18]

The clergy counselor needs to know if the NICU physicians make it a practice, as do Klaus and Kennell, to meet for counseling with parents after their infant dies. They meet with parents three times: (1) right after death, (2) two or three days after death, and (3) three to six months after the death. The main purpose of the meeting is to help the parents grieve and accept the mourning as normal. The parents can get reassurance that they are not going crazy because they cannot sleep, eat well, or seem to get anything done. If it is not the practice of physicians to meet, the clergy counselor and lay visitors, especially those who themselves have lost infants, can call pastorally on the parents for this purpose. The clergy counselor should refer the parents back to their physicians if they are suffering physical symptoms that need medical attention. The clergy should refer the parents especially if they are holding a grudge against the physicians or hospital concerning the death of the infant. Someone may have been insensitive and offended them. They may not really understand the cause of death. Law suits about "who is to blame" for the death can follow months of pent-up anger and resistance to the feelings of mourning. Sensitive physicians will welcome the chance to learn from the parent's experience.

At some point in the grieving process, if parents do not help one another accept the reality of the loss and the fact that nothing will bring back what they had hoped for, they will need help that challenges the excessive *self-centeredness* of prolonged or pathological grief. This problem can particularly affect those who do not "give in" to the need to mourn and miss the point of what is happening to them by excessive busyness or the appearance of normality when they return home from the hospital. Sadness, loneliness, and despair are feelings that most men have been taught are to be avoided in the interest of being "manly." Without them, however, it is not likely that the process of restoration of new life and hope can lead to new life plans. When nothing else will help grieving parents accept the loss, a clergy counselor can urge that they ask God to help them, in the words of prayer addressed directly to God. In my experience, personal prayer should only be used when nothing else will strengthen them for the task of "letting go" of their injured self and believing that life is good enough to continue living.

If the cause of death stemmed from a genetic disorder, and the couple plan to have another child, the clergy counselor needs to know if they received adequate genetic counseling about risks of reproduction while in the hospital. If not, a referral can be made at this time. In areas of the country that are at some distance from genetic counseling, the parents must travel to a geneticist. If the couple plans to use prenatal diagnosis with the planned new pregnancy, the clergy counselor could be asked for help with any moral or ethical problems the couple perceive. This possibility leads into the substance of the next chapter, counseling in the context of moral problems.

A Footnote on Physicians' Attitudes Toward Death

In my experience, death in a NICU or in any unit of a hospital is an opening for clergy to be faithful companions to physicians. Physicians suffer greatly when a patient dies, but many never "let on" about it. Physicians are inculcated with the belief that death is failure and that they must fight it off to the end. As Fox and Swazey comment: "Whatever nuanced attitudes towards death medical educators may intend to convey, the core conception they actually impart is that the physician is the guardian of life and adversary of death."[19] An invitation to have a cup of coffee and look back on what happened can be an opportunity for the physician to talk about the experience of losing a patient and what can be learned from it spiritually. After coming to know David Abramson, a neonatalogist who used such opportunities, I asked him to let me record and publish his reflections on the development of his own attitude about death. As I now look at this material, first transcribed in 1974, I see the distinct outlines of the religious process at work in the formation of his attitude.

This whole subject was carefully avoided in training . . . but when I look back on the past ten years, I can see an evolution in myself and the way I relate to patients. At first, I thought that death was the enemy, and that my job as a doctor was to fight it and avoid it as much as medical science gave me power to do so. When I was a resident, I began for the first time to participate in decisions to turn off the respirator, but I did it with a sense that death was inevitable, and I could reluctantly accept it when I could not do anymore to stop it.

This I feel was a compromise with death. The change in me began when I started having trouble and being anxious in relating to parents with very sick newborns. I couldn't sleep very well and was at times terrified by the decisions I had to make. I began therapy and my eyes were opened that it was fear of my own death that was frightening me and getting in my way with the parents. I began to change when I was able to accept the fact that I, too, am going to die.

Now I actually see that death is desirable for some babies, and I can face the decision in myself that I want this particular baby to die, that it is valid and a good outcome for me to work towards. I learned that I could not make good decisions about death until I had accepted death as a part of life. I can come out from behind my professional role and share in the anger and loss of giving up to death. I could not do that earlier.[20]

5. Counseling in Moral Dilemmas Caused by Applied Human Genetics

The purpose of this chapter is to recapture the moral experience of those who need and give guidance in the dilemmas of applied human genetics. A dilemma is a situation that involves a choice between equally unsatisfying alternatives. A moral dilemma is a situation in which one can appeal to moral rules and ethical principles for support of either alternative.

Clergy are expected to be competent in giving moral and ethical guidance. As more and more people participate in applied human genetics, more clergy will want to be informed about the types of moral problems that are associated with screening, prenatal diagnosis, and prospects for therapy.

I distinguish between moral and ethical guidance. To give moral guidance is to seek a resolution of a specific moral dilemma or problem. To give ethical guidance is to help clarify the special kind of reasoning that we are expected to do about moral choices, namely, reasoning supported by ethical principles that carry great weight in shaping what is considered in "the best interests" of individuals and the society itself. When clergy are asked to help with a moral problem, one or more persons present themselves with a concrete problem that is a conflict of interests. Attached to the resolution of moral problems is an obligation to explain the reasoning that we used or are to use in deciding for or against the options. One is not considered a responsible adult until he or she can engage in ethical arguments to support a moral choice.

The moral counsel provided by clergy exceeds the more customary goals of the moral guide or teacher of ethics. Clergy are expected to venture "behind" ethics, into the territory called *metaethics,* and ask troubling questions like "Where does morality come from?" or "Why should we be moral at all?" or "Is ethics sufficient to hold the human self together in the face of the terrors of life?" They are also expected to give plausible answers to these universal questions. The commitments of the human heart that underlie the institutions of morality and various systems of ethics are the special territory of the clergy. Clergy are expected to be faithful companions to others who venture out and challenge what is to many forbidden territory, namely, the prevailing *mores* of the society. Because physicians, scientists, and parents themselves have ventured out to the edges of the *mores* in the activities of applied human genetics, their dilemmas are especially revealing of the religious process that emerges in the pressures, tensions, successes, and failures of moral deliberations. When the religious process is faithfully followed in moral and ethical problems, the conventional morality is tested by human needs and the insufficiency of moral codes to deliver a "right answer."

Beginnings in Moral Experience

I have been involved professionally in many medical situations where moral choices have had to be made. These choices typically occur when:

- parents and physicians face a decision to treat or not to treat a newborn with a serious disease
- families and physicians struggle with a decision of whether and how to tell a patient the truth about the diagnosis and its implications
- parents face a decision about ending a wanted pregnancy after prenatal diagnosis of a genetic disease in the fetus
- scientists feel the shock of ethical controversy about the use of recombinant DNA for treatment of disease or fertilizing human eggs with sperm under laboratory conditions.

How do we know that we are in a moral problem? The first hint comes from the feelings and emotions we experience in the beginnings of the story of the problem.

The doorway to moral experience is conflict, contradiction, or a choice that "terrifies," as the neonatalogist, David Abramson, described it in the account of his education as a physician. My own recollection of beginnings in such situations is of how much the participants, including myself, resemble the parents of children born with a serious disease. *Numbness* and riveting attention to *detail* also mark us when we first step through the doorway of a moral problem. Something unchosen and unwanted is happening. No human being goes looking for moral problems. There is conflict in the air. Something is being born that makes us uneasy.

Yet, if we had a videotape of ourselves in the earliest stages of a moral problem, it would be hard to tell that anything important is going on. People appear detached and talk in low, controlled voices. What they are likely to talk about are the details. What the clergy hear first is the diagnosis, the circumstances of the situation, and how things might have been different (the "if onlys"). In a medical context, I have noticed in myself and other clergy a tendency to "play doctor" by asking people questions about the medical details and thus encouraging a false start in ministry. Clergy have no special competence to understand a diagnosis. Their task is first of all to help the persons who ask them for guidance to understand the terms of asking for and giving help. "For what do you want my help?" is the salient question.

What happens in the beginnings of moral dilemmas? I see first how the forms of passivity cloak and mask the conflicts that arise between what different individuals want or between conflicting desires in one individual. The most serious threat to good companionship in the beginnings of a moral problem is that the companion-to-be will be numb to the play and counterplay of forces and interests at work in the situation. Not to be trapped too soon on one of the horns of the dilemma (also read "set of self-interests") is the art form that is required. For example, in the case of Mr. and Mrs. T. in Chapter 4, if we really were to be fair to the parents, Dr. L. and I would have included them in the deliberations and been more honest about our genuine disagreement with their reasoning. Talking passively about fairness is one thing. Being fair by actions is another.

Each new occasion for companionship begins with feelings about the people, the problems, and the choices posed in the situation. The first rule of companionship is to be honest with yourself about your own feelings and emotions. You need not always disclose these to others, especially when they act in a way that shows they are unreceptive to a disclosure. But if companions are not to lose the way in the beginning, we need to be honest with ourselves about what goes on within us when troubled people consult us for ethical or religious guidance. The companion needs to give him or herself the bread of reality.

It is difficult to begin when everyone, including the companion, is numb. What is passivity? Erikson described it as a state of "inactivation of the ego,"[1] the problem-solving, observing dimension of the psyche. Passivity means that we disengage from responses already begun. People in the situation are already responding to the problem at hand with certain feelings or emotions, but they evade the responsibility to speak about these in the first person singular. Mr. and Mrs. T. talked about what would be in the interest of the child rather than in their interest. The root meaning of the word "to sin" is to miss the point or to evade. Evasion that results in self-deception is Public Enemy Number One in being a faithful companion in moral deliberations.

There are three good reasons why clergy need to help those in moral trouble notice their feelings as the relationship begins. First, it is a good opportunity to test oneself and the others. The companion-to-be needs to know something of his or her inner resources with these people. And there is also a need to know what the others' personal resources are. If they cannot or will not talk about their feelings a different kind of help, perhaps psychiatric, is needed. Only a small risk is involved in saying something like, "Would you be interested in my feelings and observations?"

The second reason is that this step is insurance against unacknowledged feelings, like anger or confusion, being the reason for sabotage of the relationship in the future. Asking for help makes us angry because of the experience of helplessness. No one purely enjoys asking for help. Besides, the situation they are in is enough to make them angry. People also are easily confused about the role of the clergy in times of trouble. Stereotypes can be at work, such as the one of the clergyperson who will pray and leave. Perhaps other clergy have left a bad taste in the mouth for religious work. The time must be taken to explore these perceptions.

The third reason is inherent in the nature of religious guidance. As long as we stay on the surface of things and take no risks to go deeper, the religious process cannot begin. Since religion means to "go behind," it happens often that the first task is to get behind the numbness and obsession with details of those who are in trouble. The first step of the journey can be to go through the door of the way the people actually behave. The bread of reality, in the beginnings of religious work, needs be offered to fill the hunger for reality behind the suppressed and bruised feelings of people who can join readily in the tasks of responsibility that lie ahead, if they are helped to take the chance. If we try to be safe and "nondirective" in the beginning, we may figuratively lose our lives.

By way of practicing this point and reviewing the dynamics of asking and being asked for moral and religious guidance, let us examine briefly how we might feel in the places of the clergy or parents described in the cases in Chapter 1. I can speak only for myself.

First, there is a real wish in me that these kinds of demands never appear, or that they disappear quickly. Why do people show up with such insoluble problems? I fear that they will blame me no matter what the outcome. But I chose the kind of work that invites people in trouble to present themselves. I have to remind myself that I do have the choice to do something else and that the real purpose of religion is to serve people who do not "have it made."

Secondly, as I enter each case again or for the first time, I am aware of many conflicting desires, loyalties, and duties. There is the pull of an obligation to be truthful, even to fourteen-year-old girls at risk for Huntington's disease (Case 1), as well as to a grown man whose wife and physician are deceiving him (Case 2). On the other side, there is the pull to protect the girl and her younger sister from possible psychological harm. Or is that my own and the mother's anxiety speaking? Yes, I can understand the physician's and the wife's fear that her husband may physically hurt her and the child. But is not this physician being too protective and paternalistic by trying to take care of the marriage over and beyond the genetic risks? Who appointed him as the sole arbiter of what the husband should know?

In the case of the Protestant counselor and the Catholic mother (Case 3), I would feel caught like a fly in a trap. I am sympathetic to a fault, especially with persons with burning moral problems. I am also very sensitive (some say too much) about being cut off from colleagues in my profession from another denomination. If I respond to her and see her alone, I am only asking for trouble from a priest who has a pastoral relationship with her. If I do not respond to her, and see her on her own terms, I risk the chance that she will have no one to talk with. Also, there is the fate of the child-to-be, the affected fetus she is carrying, to consider.

In Case 4, I am aware of a need to help the physician complete her responsibility to the grieving parents, and I am also aware that the parents did not ask for the pastor's help. Should clergy meet with anyone under these conditions? I appreciate the risk of being unpopular with a physician whose organization helps pay the bills. I will lose self-respect if I meet with literally anyone on any terms at all. Then there is the guilt I would feel if I contributed to the birth of yet another child with paralysis if I did not respond to the physician.

In the case of Dr. Cline, the doctor who attempted experimental gene therapy, I first feel vindictive. He got what was coming to him for breaking the rules so willfully. On the other side, I know what it means to want to be "first," especially when one might do good for others at the same time. I can also identify with his frustration at having his plans blocked by a committee of peers, but his actions were not justified.

These are feelings, composed of complex bundles of emotions and beliefs piling in one on the other. Sorting them out is one thing. I love to sort and analyze things, peeling one layer from another to see what is next. I can even enjoy watching myself work in this kind of analytical stance. The trouble starts when I ask myself, as well as those to whom I am responsible, "what are your truest feelings, most prized beliefs, or most cherished values in this mix of things? Who are you and can you make sense of yourself?" The beginnings of religious work are threatened by the danger that we will be overwhelmed by conflicts, or that we will be simply like chameleons who blend in with any possibility. The companion needs to be a student of emotional process to understand the links of emotion to belief. But since we ought not make moral decisions merely on the strength of emotions alone, the next problem is posed by the question, "What ought I do in this situation?" A moral choice must be made.

Moral Guidance: What Ought I or We Do in This Situation?

Whenever the "ought question" is posed directly to an individual or group, there is a resultant impact or shock, if there is a conscience there to receive the question. Sociopaths are not shocked by the ought question. Nazis do not seek moral guidance. When this question arises, the experience is of being confronted from within and without.

The community has an interest in the resolution of every ought question. There are rules that have evolved to apply to moral conflicts. Moral rules like "be fair," "be truthful," "don't cause harm," "do not kill," and the like remind us that when another's welfare is at stake in the conflict, the welfare of all will be involved in the example set by the resolution to the conflict. Moral problems involve conflicts of competing interests, desires, or values. To the extent that we have internalized the rules that apply to the particular conflict, we will feel their impact.

Also, to the degree that we are good companions to ourselves, we will ask what the relevance of the rules is to the particular situation, test for exceptions, and generally treat ourselves as if we had enough autonomy to weigh the matter for ourselves. Weighing what the community expects against what we desire, and sifting the cost and promise of the alternatives that emerge, is what we do at first in moral deliberations.

What, however, are you supposed to do when two very good rules conflict, as in the case of the deceived husband (Case 2)? It is a good thing to tell the truth, and it is also good to protect persons from harm. By what technique will I break the deadlock between the choices? Either way, the people involved will lose something. I get anxious because I cannot forsee the many consequences that will attach to my choice and accumulate for years to come. Who can really count the cost of taking the risk to confront a wife and a physician with their well-meaning deception? Who can really count the cost to one's self-respect of playing the game with them?

There is another layer of complexity in the experience of being asked by a person in need, "What is the church's mind on this issue?" This question frequently arises about abortion. The problem is that the churches are often of two or three minds. There is disagreement about morality. Additionally, we live in a society in which no one has a monopoly on moral truth. If I, as a moral guide, consult the most respected writings in moral philosophy, I find no final agreement about what is in people's best moral interests. Some think it means to do the most good for those in the situation and others similarly situated, defining good in terms of measurable benefits. Others think that to be good means to avoid acts that are intrinsically evil (in their view), such as lying, no matter what the consequences. As I consider the question, "Should a therapeutic lie be condoned?" many moral injunctions make demands upon my conscience. For example:

- "Do not let a day pass before the full truth can be known, even at the risk of danger."
- "Obey your self-interest and restrain your need to help; leave the decision completely to her."
- "See to it that the truth is never known, because the chances of personal harm are too great."
- "Advise her to ask her husband to come into counseling with her, so that the groundwork can be laid for telling him all at a later date."

No one injunction perfectly satisfies the good things that might be accomplished or restrains all of the destructive possibilities. No injunction satisfies all of the duties involved.

As I struggle with the issue of who will be right or wrong, three problems about morality raise their heads. The first is the inevitability of decisions. Even a decision to avoid a decision is a decision.

The one thing I cannot avoid is to decide. The second problem is that one called heteronomy and autonomy. I shall never satisfy the need to please the panels of moral experts in my head, and I shall never make a decision if I continue to try to please them. Closure on the problem means to decide it. But I feel that I must make a decision that makes moral sense and that fits into the ways and rules of the moral community whose values I most espouse. Yet I must make a decision that I can square with my own need for self-respect and independence. There is no solution to this tension, apparently, and it clouds the decision with admixtures of coloration that are disturbing.

The third problem is in the nature of a decision. I am reminded that the word comes from *decidare,* a root meaning "to cut off." To decide means to cut off alternatives that I shall not have or enjoy. In addition to the anxiety about being wrong or confused in moral choice, there is a feeling of sadness and loss about the alternatives that I decide against, especially those that I imagine later would have turned out for the best. What would have happened *if* is another of those disturbing questions that provokes our solitude and invokes the "is it worth it?" question. T. S. Eliot may have had the same feeling in mind when he wrote these lines:

> Footfalls echo in the memory
> Down the passage which we did not take
> Towards the door we never opened
> Into the rose-garden.[2]

Then I commit myself and make a decision or a series of decisions. By venturing out, I lose what is left behind. If I do not venture out and decide, I suffer a loss of a very serious kind. I erase myself and disappear as a person. Grieving over the losses brought about by passivity has driven many people to seek the help of clergy. If I do make the decision and commit myself, I notice that I can grieve over the losses of the alternatives that are gone forever. Then a new kind of problem can set in. I feel that I must explain my decisions to others or, even worse, I feel that I must justify the decisions and myself on a figurative witness stand before an all-knowing audience. The endless circles and self-righteousness of the process of justification are appalling. Are we so different, my reader and myself ?

Before passing on to the issues of ethical guidance, let me tell you where I come out on the cases in Chapter 1 involving moral guidance.

Case 1: Who Is Too Young for Genetic Counseling?

I favor encouraging the mother to take the girls to a genetic counselor, with their father, even though the marriage has ended. The girls are entitled to the same information that those who can read a newspaper can learn for themselves. The father is the affected member of the family and the girls should hear from him how it is living with the knowledge. Additionally, the more people who know that they are at risk, the greater the likelihood that pressure will build for scientists and physicians to find a reliable method of diagnosis and treatment.

Case 2: Should a Therapeutic Lie Be Condoned?

I favor calling the physician to arrange for a meeting to take place in his office. Present should be physician, wife, husband, and pastor. I would also recommend that a psychiatrist be consulted in planning the meeting. He or she would also be present to evaluate the potential for physical danger and, in any event, make recommendations for the well-being of the couple and child. The physician has knowledge to which a patient, the husband, is entitled. The physician's duty, however painful, is to inform the husband that he is at risk for being a carrier. The physician is in legal as well as moral jeopardy by having already contacted the wife separately. If the husband discovers that he has been deceived, he will have a good case of negligence against the physician. The marriage may end, but the husband will need to know his true genetic status if he plans to remarry. If the physician refused to hold the meeting, I would say that the new code of ethics of the American Medical Association requires that a physician who deals dishonestly with patients be reported to the local medical society. Does the physician seriously want me to see to it that this is done? I would also consider calling the physician over the objections of the wife, because if the husband found out that I had been told and did nothing to interrupt the deception, he could well take out his fury physically on the pastor, rather than the wife, if he is indeed at risk for committing homicide. For this and other reasons, I do not automatically say to people in trouble that I will always "keep a confidence." I ask them to risk telling me what the confidence is and then let me make the decision whether or not to keep it.

Case 3: Consequences of a Sex-Linked Disorder

The pastoral counselor made an error of judgment, in my view. The counselor could have spent more time on the phone and found out what the situation involved, rather than commit to a meeting. I favor offering her the chance for a meeting with four people involved: the husband, the priest, herself, and the counselor, if she wants help with the communication issues with the priest. If the priest turns her down, the Protestant counselor should then see her. The priest will certainly find out that she had an abortion, if she goes through with her intention. Perhaps she cannot live with the idea of abortion and is looking for a way out, namely, to have someone else besides a priest suggest that she go to term with pregnancy and try again. She could also consider allowing the child to be adopted. I would not preempt her right to decide for herself on the abortion issue, but I would not neglect the opportunity to be a mediator between her family and the priest.

Case 4: Who Is the Pastor to Help?

I favor the idea of a meeting with physician and parents, but I would ask the physician to have the father ask me for a meeting. Even poor mountaineers can sense that a physician is out of line by talking with a pastor about their problems without consulting them first. Besides, the couple does not belong to the pastor's congregation. The pastor should be cautious about having the authority of his office used to promote genetic counseling. I also favor his telling the physician that his position in the meeting will be to see that the parents have all the facts, learn all the options, and explore the consequences. She should advocate screening if she feels strongly about it, but the pastor should not. If the parents decide to refuse screening and complete the pregnancy, the pastor should be prepared to help them with the problems that will arise if the new child also has a neural tube defect. If they decide to accept screening and in the event the pregnancy is terminated by abortion, the pastor should be prepared to help them with problems that arise with this choice as well.

A Pattern of Moral Guidance

Methods of giving moral guidance differ as widely as theological views on the proper authority and role of the clergy. Some examples include (1) the assignment of the penance in the context of oral confession; (2) the rabbinic interpretation of the requirement of Jewish law; (3) officially adopted reports of experts on certain moral problems by a religious body; (4) the "teaching sermon" about a moral problem that ends with the clergyperson taking a position; and (5) exploration of a moral problem in the context of "pastoral counseling," followed by leaving the decisions to the conscience of the believer. Clergy can be involved in each of these patterns of guidance.

For the first ten years of my pastoral practice, I tended to give moral guidance from the pulpit and in the counseling room. My method was largely "nondirective," like my premarital counseling. I would help the other (congregation or person) identify the moral problem, explore its implications, and leave the matter "open" for their decision. I made exceptions to this general position for social issues that my denomination's elected leaders discussed in official statements of guidance.

I have adopted a different method of giving moral guidance that possibly reflects my experiences in applied bioethics, but there are parallels to the clergy role. Physicians expect nondirective moral guidance, probably because they compare the process of asking for moral guidance with the tradition of using a medical consultant.

Problems can arise in the care of a patient that cause the physician to ask for the opinion of a specialist. The specialist then takes on the role of "medical consultant." The consultant studies the problem, makes a recommendation, and then steps aside. The attending physician has the responsibility for the proper use of the recommendation. If the consultant knows that the physician has not followed the recommendation, he or she cannot override the decision because the patient belongs to the attending physician.

The crucial difference between being a medical consultant and a consultant in moral dilemmas is the possibility that one or more resolutions are offensive to the consultant's values, or (even more difficult) when a particular resolution breaks rules or guidelines of the consultant's institution. If Dr. Cline (Case 5) had consulted me about his dilemma as to whether to attempt gene therapy in patients even though it would have violated the rules of protection of human subjects, I would have recommended that he wait until more animal research proved the value of trying in humans. If he "confided" in me that he planned a trip to other nations to do this trial, I would not have felt bound by this communication and also warned him that if he did so, I would report his intentions to the authorities. If he did not heed the warning, I would have reported him.

The consultant in a moral dilemma cannot simply "step aside" from the recommendation. Of course, clergy and other counselors can avoid getting into this dilemma by not making any recommendation at all. I wonder if the real function of nondirective counseling and moral guidance is to help the counselor never get into the dilemma of "What ought I do if the proposed resolution itself is morally unacceptable?" If you never make any recommendations, then you never have to face the question, except in your own conscience.

I was pushed into taking a more active role in giving moral counsel by the fact that my institution has a highly developed set of rules to protect human subjects in research. If I am asked for counsel by a physician-investigator in a dilemma about a matter that also involves these rules, I must make it clear that my counsel is not value-free. If the one seeking counsel intends to proceed in violation of the rules, I must call on higher authority to help resolve the problem in some satisfactory way. If I did not, then I would be involved in a type of conspiracy and would be undermining the purpose of my work, namely, to assure that the rules of the institution are respected. The rules are constantly "in process," evolving, being changed to adapt to new circumstances, but these rules help make research possible in our complex, free society in which it is morally objectionable to coerce persons in any way to be research subjects.

There are higher values than the good that can be done by research, even when the good can be life-saving.

Are not the clergy in a similar position to mine *vis a vis* the moral traditions and preferences of the religious bodies? Every denomination has a body of moral practices, rules, and traditions that it cherishes. Family life, marriage, parenthood, and human reproduction comprise some, but not all, of the matters of responsibility that the moral traditions of religious bodies address. Let us suppose that a married member of a congregation consults its clergyperson about the moral dilemma of whether to end a marriage and begin a new relationship with another person, also married, that could lead to what is believed to be a "happier marriage" for both. It emerges that the seeker of guidance has already had sexual relations with the other married person and plans to continue seeing that person. And suppose the clergyperson had officiated at both marriages. If the clergyperson is nondirective and leaves the dilemma with the one who seeks help, what happens to the integrity of the tradition of monogamous marriage and the commandment about adultery in his or her religious body? If the clergyperson acts in a way that demeans respect for the moral tradition, how can anyone else be expected to uphold it? Some laity may expect nondirective moral guidance because of the strong bias towards individualism in American religion or because the religious body itself puts the highest value on freedom of conscience. But I believe that the moral issue for the clergy as guides to others will not go away. There is a price to pay for being in the role of a clergyperson that we avoid to our detriment and to the detriment of our denominations.

I have changed the beginning of a consultation with another who asks for moral guidance to include an element of the "informed consent" process. Typically, I will receive a call from someone who wants to see me or talk then about a problem. If possible, I try not to talk on the telephone, unless it is an emergency. The caller usually says that a matter or a problem "is worrying me." I ask the caller to make an appointment to see me in private. In the meeting, before the person tells me the substance of the concern, I introduce myself and sketch the outlines of my job. I let the person know that if the consultation requires keeping a matter confidential that is related to my central concern (i.e., the protection of human subjects in research), I will not agree beforehand to do it. I ask them if they want to proceed with this understanding, they may also take the risk of letting me decide about whether to keep the matter confidential. I add that if they want my help in resolving the problem, I cannot guarantee them that it will not come to the attention of others, including those in authority. Thus far, I have not seen anyone unwilling to proceed. Probably, when they cross the threshhold of asking for help in the first place, they are uncomfortable enough with the problem to have little difficulty in accepting these terms.

After I hear the person out, I study the problem from as many angles as possible. If more information is needed to answer questions that I cannot answer, I wait until further information is in. I then make a recommendation about one or more resolutions that I favor, with reasons as to why these and not others are acceptable. Most of the time, people who consult me can carry out the needed action themselves. It has happened, however, that my help and the help of others in authority were needed to resolve the problem.

By analogy, every clergyperson has a "central concern" of his or her responsibility. Ordination vows in each denomination frame the general requirements of the clergy role. Services of installation of clergy in congregations frame specific expectations to safeguard the integrity of the tradition as expressed in the life of the congregation. As was discussed in Chapter 2, the majority of laity expect clergy to be persons of integrity. In my view, we let them down when we are so nondirective as to risk minimal involvement by making no recommendations at all in moral problems.

Ethical Guidance

Ethics is a complex term that points to a content and a process.[3] The content of ethics is composed of foundational principles, moral rules, and concepts that shape ideal portraits of the moral life of the individual and the best interests of the society. Ethics is also a process with several purposes in addition to depiction of ideal states of being. Ethics has an *educative* purpose. To know ourselves even as we act and decide is in itself a moral imperative. We are expected to become more self-knowledgable by examination of past and future decisions. Ethics also has a *social* purpose, in that ethical questions and issues are construed on a level of impartiality and generality.

When we "raise" ethical questions, what we really do is try to move the conflict to a level removed from personal and ideological bias. Without this push, or view from above, conflicts remain embroiled in sheer emotion or polarization. Ethics also presses towards a *religious* purpose, because our motivation and inspiration to want to be moral at all is drawn from sources that lie in the territory known as *metaethics,* beyond the bodies of principles and rules that comprise the ethical systems.

To my mind, ethics is best understood as a conceptual process with a goal of accountability. You can see the process at work on the individual and social levels. We engage in extended conversations with ourselves about "was that decision really right?" What follows in the mind, if it is ethical reflection, is critical examination of the reasons we gave to support the decisions. Were these the best reasons? If a moral rule or set of guidelines was involved in the press of decision, we may go back mentally and explore whether the rule was applicable or relevant especially if someone eloquently objected to your interpretation. When we make choices, we should expect to hear questions within ourselves about them. If not, there is danger abroad in the self.

When we give answers to the "ought" question, we should expect that our answers will be answered by others responsible for critical examination of what is in the best interests of individuals and society. Ethics is a social process of answering the "ought" question and being answered by others who have authority to evaluate your answer. Authority figures in ethics are to be found in the professions, in universities, in literature and the arts, and in religious bodies. But there is an authority in every person that legitimates any question about the appropriateness of the reasons given for moral choice as well as whether the moral codes themselves are adequate. Morality is socially produced and is evaluated in the ethical process. You are not considered a responsible adult until you can engage in reasoning about the decisions you make.

The function of accountability, the goal of the ethical process, is that we learn the strengths and weaknesses of the reasons we advance to support the choices that we make. Can we recommend the reasoning that we used to others who are similarly situated? Just making a choice is not sufficient. One is expected to give reasons and, if it is a moral choice, to show how ethical principles shape and support the choice. The word "principle" is from the Latin *principium* or "beginning." Ethical principles, rather than egoistic interests or expediency, must be the point of departure in ethical argument or else the process breaks down. Ethical principles coalesce beliefs and values for which persons would be willing to sacrifice any comfort or convenience. Under oppressive conditions or when the basic principles of the institutions of the society are threatened, people are willing to die to preserve principles. Some of the ethical principles that shape assumptions about institutions in this society are justice, veracity, beneficience, nonmaleficence, autonomy, equality, and utility.

We should expect to be answered back by those who detect weaknesses in our moral reasoning. Weaknesses can be of several sorts. An argument can be fallacious in terms of logic. It can be circular, simply demonstrating the premise but leading to no conclusion. It can be self-serving or ideological, masking the interests of a group or profession. A moral argument can be based on conflicting principles or be too confused to recommend to others. The critic may show that the premise on which the argument is based is itself unethical in the light of principles for which humans are willing to die, or at least sacrifice very much.

Having been heard and answered, you are then expected to reconsider the choice and the argument supporting the choice. If the argument is weak, the proper thing to do is to admit it and show how it can be strengthened. If, in the light of criticism, you believe you made the wrong choice, you can change your position without blame. You are also expected to be grateful for criticism.

To give and receive ethical guidance is a form of human activity that occurs, necessarily, at a stage removed from the conflict and heat of decisions. Universities, seminar rooms, official commissions, and high-level conferences are the most prominent locales of the give-and-take of the ethical process. Books, essays, and articles are media of the dialogue. In religious bodies, the sermon, pastoral letter, or encyclical are frequently employed to reach the level of seriousness and impartiality needed for ethical judgments and considerations.

I repeat that, to my mind, the basic purpose of ethics is accountability. We are to *learn* the strengths and weaknesses of what we consider our best reasoning. And we are to keep the moral institutions for which we are responsible under constant criticism for their efficacy to illuminate and facilitate the resolution of moral conflicts. Moral institutions are bodies of norms, standards, rules, and guides to action to which we turn in the press of everyday life for guidance in moral problems. The ethical process is the major means by which morality is criticized, repaired, and renewed. Jesus' teaching that "the Sabbath was made for man, not man for the Sabbath" (Mark 2:27) is relevant to the distinction between the ethical process and morality. The moral or religious code is not to be treated with the absolute respect due only to God, who inspires the courage to see through institutional realities and understand them for what they are. Ethics is the process by which we hold up our decisions and moral institutions to the light of criticism inspired by the beliefs and values of the cultural traditions that we most cherish.

Does Ethics Make Sense of the Meaning of Life?

In my experience, normative arguments that begin from ethical principles do not come directly into play in the press of making decisions. Neither clergy, physicians, nor parents ask themselves which ethical theory makes the most sense of the decision. We make decisions with the help of whatever moral equipment we have acquired but, apparently, this is not enough. I imagine countless ways that I want my decision to *fit into* traditions of morality, ethics, and religion that I have studied, tried to practice, and respect. These traditions are revealed in the best and worst moments of the collective history of the people to whom I choose to belong.

There is a need to make *ethical* sense, as well as moral and emotional sense. Humans have the capacity to entertain such questions as, "Are my decisions in the best interests of others like myself? Would I want them to follow the example of my reasoning about the decision?" My experience is that there is also conflict at the ethical level and a need to make sense of challenges to the adequacy of our ethics and the principles that are supposed to guide decisions. What is consistently the most trustworthy vision of the good and moral life? What does it mean to be truly responsible as one self among all my companions on earth?

It is easy, in this society, to neglect the need to make sense of conflicts between competing ethical principles or claims made in the name of principle. Do claims for truth-telling always override all of the consequences that may result from opening a secret? Does the good that we can do always override the harm that will be done to what is right? How much weight should be given to different interpretations of what is good and right? Our society places a high value on pragmatism, a mentality committed to solving problems. "Does it work?" may be the most frequent barometer of good and evil in our time. I often question whether good money is wasted supporting philosophers who pound away at definitions of justice, rights, or what is truly the good life. I remind myself what I know beneath my skepticism. We are creatures who decide and choose, even at the level of what principles should shape our best reasoning about decisions past, present, and future. There are different spirits that compete for the honor of being the ambience at the table where decisions are made. If you prefer the image of life as a game, there are different spirits that compete for domination of the shaping of the rules and terms of the game, as well as the way disputes are settled. If I am asked what accounts for my choice of principles, I have to point to beliefs and preferences drawn from many sources, not all of them theological, about what is in the best interests of individuals and society. But the possibility of disagreements at the level of ethics is profound. A feeling of vertigo often comes over me after debates on ethics that makes me fear and doubt the value of further argument.

Ethical Systems in Human Culture

There are two major ethical systems in our culture that compete for dominance in the midst of moral problems. Technically, these approaches are called "deontological" and "teleological." Translated into ordinary language, the first approach emphasizes that certain acts are *right or wrong in themselves,* or that certain rules are intrinsically sound and should be followed virtually without exception and regardless of the consequences. The second approach is held by those who mainly look at the *goals and consequences* of the alternatives in the decision, and who concentrate on trying to promote the greatest amount of good and restrain the greatest amount of evil in the circumstances. There are many variations on these themes, but these two systems are clearly dominant contending positions defended in moral controversies. For example, the abortion debate is marked by appeals to the essential equality of all human beings that abortion violates (according to those who are opposed), and on the other side by appeals to the number of maternal lives that can be saved and tangible suffering alleviated.

"Deontological" refers to the Greek root *deont*, meaning "duty." Those who hold this position assert that the compelling forces acting on the decisionmaker are universal standards or rules inherent in nature or established through supernatural revelation. The understanding of responsibility derived from this approach is conveyed in the words "law" and "duty." An example of this approach in the realm of health is that the decisions of a physician should be guided by the inherent sanctity of human life. The preservation of life and the life process is understood to be a universal axiom.

"Teleological" refers to a root meaning "goal" or "end." Those who argue for this position stress that the most compelling factor in a decision is the goal(s) being sought. Responsibility is usually understood in this framework as a virtue or goodness brought about through the discipline of goalseeking that can be measured in tangible rather than intangible ways. In the realm of health, those who espouse this position are mainly concerned with the concrete relief or prevention of suffering.

In his writings, H. Richard Niebuhr attempted to synthesize and transcend the conflicting demands of these two systems.[4] He concentrated on the *relationship* between the responses of the decisionmaker and the forces acting upon him or her, including the influences of the demands of these two ethical systems. The responsible decisionmaker lives in a process of interaction with the surrounding forces, including the ethical demands of the culture and its forms of ethical reasoning. Niebuhr drew a lesson in ethics from the analogy of driving an automobile. If good driving is analogous to good living, what goes into good driving? There is certainly the destination (goal) and there are rules of the road (law) that we must observe. But is one or either of these the essence of driving? On the contrary, good driving involves the quality of those hundreds, even thousands, of decisions made by the driver from the beginning to the end of the trip. The total journey is a complex story in which the driver is affected by many forces, not the least being the quality and contour of the road. Among the many forces acting on the driver are the goal or destination and the traffic laws. These must be processed continuously against the background of the present dangers and opportunities of the road. Responsible living is like responsible driving. Responsibility translates into the "ability to respond" to the many forces acting upon the self in a manner that maintains the integrity of the self. To be unable to respond, to evade action, or to be overwhelmed by the many different demands of decisions, is to find oneself in moral confusion. There is some moral confusion in every decision that makes us anxious about the conflicts. Moral confusion can escalate into a total state of confusion, sometimes called *anomie*, a terrible state of drifting normlessness.

Another experience of conflict and anxiety arises when I ask myself, "Well, why be moral anyway? Everyone looks out for themselves first and I know it, so why shouldn't I?" Does it make sense to strive to do the good and the right thing when the actions of so many make a mockery of ethics? There are other versions of the same suspicion, such as the maxim that "morality begins at the end of the barrel of a gun." What can uphold me when even the premise of being moral at all can be so much in doubt?

Does not death itself have the final word on all our strivings, including the moral kind? The point is that not even ethical principles, in themselves, furnish the final sources of self-respect and respect for others required to make morality and ethics possible at all. Without a source of commitment "beyond ethics" that nurtures a spirit of reciprocity and cooperation, there could be no common life. This recognition is the beginning of religious experience for many people, namely, that there is a need for a source of guidance that holds together when morality itself can be radically questioned. Indeed, when I am honest with myself, morality is continually open to question.

The clergy, physicians, and parents in the case studies are filled with conflicting loyalties, desires, and goals. If we put ourselves in their place, which is the purpose of the exercise of case studies, we know that in such situations we will reflect our need to be account- able to others who share our loyalties. We will feel pressure, per- haps anger, and moral confusion. In reality, there are many conflicting pressures upon us, including many sources of ethical guidance. How can we make sense of the cacaphony of voices and pressures? How can we respond and be responsible in the midst of so many demands? This question, in my view, is the beginning of the religious process in the context of ethics. Responsibility means the decisionmaker's ability to respond to many sources of action upon him or her, including multiple sources of ethical guidance. The term "ability to respond" is complex and has several dimen- sions.

Our ability to make responses is grounded in our physical and genetic inheritance. Our ability to make *human* responses is ground- ed in the way the structures of our physical, genetic, and cultural inheritance interact with our freedom, that which makes us unique- ly human. The quality of freedom that marks us as human can best be understood as the quality of the "openness" of the world of humans. A dog's world is "closed" in the sense that it can only patrol the outer limits of what has been laid down by the instincts as modified by training. A mouse's world is even more closed than a dog's, at least territorially. The human world is open in the sense that it can both be imagined differently and modified far beyond the limits of any of the given structures that help us to navigate that world. The quality of freedom extends not only to the physical changes that can be brought about in the world, but also to changes in thoughts and feelings. We can revise our interpretations of the meaning of the world and the universe in which our planet is a small part.

Our ability to respond is stabilized and organized within the *struc- tures* of human culture. We are born unfinished to an extraordinary degree. The traditions, institutions, morality, and values that form our culture interact to produce the structures within which our emotions and energies are organized and directed. Religion is also one of these structures, functioning largely to protect culture's sta- bility and order. Our genetic inheritance is one of the most important, if not the most important, structures for guiding the human response. We are born as the latest point in the long story of evolution, prepared to adapt to the world and to change it.

We never exist apart from these structures, yet the sum total of all of the structures does not completely define us nor does it circumscribe our responses. There is the possibility of freedom in human responses that sets us apart in the world as we presently know it. The heart of ethics is the search for guidance in the proper use of our freedom to maintain or modify the world and ourselves, including all of the structures contained within the world. Morality is one of the structures designed to maintain and organize human energies, especially in the conflicts of individual wills and the interests of collectives. Human freedom is never so clearly demonstrated as in moral decisions and processes of change in morality. A rule or norm that is "fixed" and seen as unchanging does, in fact, change as a result of human decisions.

Our ability to respond is sustained by the structures within which we live as well as our freedom. Yet, it is possible to be richly endowed with structure and freedom and still lose the ability to respond, to fade away as a responsible person. To return for a final time to the case examples, we can picture the clergy or parents much later explaining to others what they decided, depending upon their loyalties. We can also picture them alone in the office or at home, weeping into their hands, impotent and paralyzed by the experience of many conflicts.

Most of our decisionmaking does not end in paralysis, but it can. Everyone will recognize a kind of sadness or resignation about the problem of maintaining integrity—the sense of having *one* self—in the midst of many conflicting pressures and actions. Having a different self for different occasions, one for family, one for work, one for church, one for leisure, one for politics, induces its own kind of inauthenticity and moral sickness. It turns out that our ability to respond is equally nurtured by a sense of self-respect, oneness, or integrity that holds the self together in the midst of conflicting pressure. From what source does that seed of wholeness, the source of integrity that unites the self within, really grow? What is the ground of the ability to respond that can keep me together in the midst of forces that threaten to pull me apart?

A ground of responsibility that unites the divided self is the seedbed of religion's contribution to ethics. The need for a ground of responsibility is universally shared by all humans. To be human is to make decisions. To be human is to be threatened by the anxiety of being pulled apart by irreconcilable forces in the decision. To make decisions presupposes some standpoint for *interpretation* of the meaning of decisions. We not only place a meaning upon each individual situation within which we make decisions but, if we press deeply enough, we discover that we as humans share "master interpretations" of the *whole* story of human striving and decisionmaking. We ask ourselves, "What is going on?" when confronted by conflict. What kind of a conflict is it? What is happening to me in the conflict? Beyond the habitual, instinctive kinds of decisions that do not require our creative energies, we assign interpretations to the actions upon us, and these interpretations color and condition our responses. Our sense of integrity or wholeness basically arises from the manner in which our "master interpretations" of the meaning of life interact with our day-to-day interpretations of the meaning of conflicts in which we risk our integrity or lose it. Our master interpretations include not only our beliefs about society and its institutions, our parents, and our experience with them, but an underlying and central interpretation that we place upon the *whole* of life and our part in it. There are threads that run through the fabric of our everyday responses leading back to our ultimate commitments.

The ground of responsibility for the divided self is also subject to interpretation. The one uniting action amidst all of the contending forces can be interpreted as an illusion to be foresworn, as if nothing triumphs over either death or the randomness of events in the universe. Some interpret the one action as evolutionary purpose or the cool eye of human reason. The interpretation that I hold (at times weakly, but supported by the faith of many others) is that there is one action upon us in the midst of all other actions, the God whom Jesus of Nazareth addressed as "Father." I do not believe that ethics alone provide a sufficient basis to answer the question of the meaning of responsibility. There is finally no escape from the issues posed by life's limits.

6. Counseling in Decisions After Prenatal Diagnosis

The major moral problem associated with prenatal diagnosis is elective abortion (i.e., aborting an affected fetus in the hope of having another child without the disorder). The odds of having a child without the disease are high; on the average, 96.5 percent of those who seek prenatal diagnosis receive "good news," a negative diagnosis. In about 3.5 percent of cases, the news is "bad," or a positive diagnosis. I emphasize that the diagnosis does not dictate what the couple should do. It is not automatic that, because the fetus is affected, they should choose abortion. Their views on abortion and their moral beliefs will influence what they should do. Clergy will see parents who believe that abortion is wrong and parents who are open towards abortion.

There is a moral problem at the heart of the abortion decision. On the one hand, there is the interest in the life of the fetus. On the other hand, there is the interest of the mother and the parents in protecting themselves from what they interpret to be "harm." It is good to want the fetus to live, and it is good to want to protect oneself. The conflict is deeply felt because these parents usually want a child badly. Our society is now governed by legal rules that make abortion on request legal through the second trimester, which would include the time span appropriate for prenatal diagnosis. Yet, the rules of the Supreme Court are not in themselves ethical considerations. The clergy counselor and the couple should know the arguments on both sides of the issue.

The Moral Argument Against Elective Abortion

Physicians and ethicists who have raised ethical objections against prenatal diagnosis do not attack the technique itself or express any bias toward technology. Two dominant themes appear in their arguments: (1) a basic purpose of medicine—to save life—is violated by the practice of abortion; and (2) while some abortions may be justified, the use of prenatal diagnosis tends to set apart certain fetuses as deserving of abortion and thus treats fetuses unequally and unjustly.

The critics of elective abortion may base their arguments in theologically derived beliefs, biological observations, rights based on natural law, or other philosophical considerations. However, each argument tends to come to rest in an acknowledgment of human rights and a dignity that is beyond arbitrary control.

The strongest features of the arguments against elective abortion of defective fetuses are the same as the strongest features of any arguments against abortion for any reason: the clarity and meaning that derive from (1) the unavoidable objective reality of the fetus; (2) the equality of fundamental human rights; and (3) the moral belief that personhood is immeasurable and traceable to some value that transcends the individual. The experience of being transcended by sources of meaning and dignity beyond oneself is profoundly reassuring and provides a powerful imperative for consistency rather than relativity in moral reasoning.

The strengths of this position include (1) the protection afforded to every disabled life by the principle of equality; (2) the compassion toward the individual fetus regardless of its handicap; and (3) the consistency of moral judgments applied to cases ranging from severe to minor handicaps. The weaknesses of the position derive from what is excluded from a place of overriding importance: (1) the possibility that the physical and mental problems of the infant will be an overall detriment to the mother, the family, and the resources of the society; and (2) the possibility that allowing the fetus to live will do great injury to the future child.

Arguments for Elective Abortion

The main arguments for elective abortion grow out of (1) the obligation to reduce or prevent suffering for the affected family, the fetus in question, and society; and (2) the obligation to prevent genetic disease and its impact on future generations in the absence of successful genetic therapies.

Physicians measure injury and suffering to the fetus by severity of the disease, age of onset, mortality, morbidity, presence or absence of chronic pain, mental retardation, and disfigurement. They frequently argue that the degree of suffering for the infant will be directly related to the problems presented for the family, and the two should not be separated. Rarely, it is argued, should elective abortion be done for the sake of prevention of suffering of the child. Most proponents of elective abortion reason from the relief of suffering to the parents and siblings that will be caused by the disease.

The strengths of the argument for elective abortion are that it favors (1) the enhancement of human responsibility to control the consequences of reproduction; (2) an increase in the sphere of freedom for affected families; (3) a reduction of human suffering and genetic harm; and (4) the protection of society's resources. The weaknesses of the position are related to what it rejects: (1) biological data about the individuality of the fetus are subordinated to difficult social concepts of personhood; (2) the denial of human status to the developing fetus tends to create precedents in moral reasoning for denying the right to life to other deficient, disabled, or dying persons; and (3) the position does not adequately account for the many examples of the transcendence of birth defects by individuals and families.

I agree more with the arguments that favor elective abortion than with those opposed to it, as the reader will surely have noted in previous sections. But, because I respect so highly the efforts of ethicists and religious leaders who confront society with the moral and intellectual meaning of abortion, which does kill the fetus, I not only present their views but respond to certain competing ethical claims in recommendations for a social policy on elective abortion and in counseling couples who face decisions after prenatal diagnosis. Clergy and members of congregations have influence in social policy formation and should make their views known, since abortion is an important social problem requiring resolution at the highest level of government.

Counseling in Decisions After Prenatal Diagnosis

It is crucial that the counselor and the couple respond to the abortion option as *one among several* options available. Nothing diminishes human freedom more unnecessarily than to avoid the burden of choice. In the medical realm, it is easy to fall into the fallacy that the diagnosis dictates the choice (i.e., the diagnosis is Down syndrome, therefore the conclusion is abortion). The preservation of options is also crucial for the continuing work required in society to pursue goals of curing genetic disease through research and experimentation. We must not accept elective abortion as the only social response to genetic disease in the fetus. The decisionmaking of each couple is also related to the developing social policy on elective abortion and applied human genetics. Individual and social action must be seen in the same framework.

Moral action is response to action upon us. The decision about abortion is a response to forces at work upon the couple and their counselor. First, there is an impact of *emotional* significance. The couple has just found out that they are among the 3.5 percent who get bad news. Many of the same feelings emerge as when a child is born with the disease in question. They are numb, then questioning, then angry. They may have been predisposed to abortion before entering genetic counseling, and they will have talked about it with one another earlier. However, when they receive news of the positive diagnosis, in effect, they must make the decision anew. At this point, they may ask help from a clergyperson. The wise clergy will have been following the couple all along. People in the abortion decision suffer emotionally and morally. They wanted to have a healthy baby enough to go through the long wait for amniocentesis (sixteen to eighteen weeks), and they waited an agonizing three additional weeks for the lab work to be done. They learned about the diagnosis from the geneticist-physician on the phone or in person. They may question the accuracy of the finding or the physician's abilities. There is also fear about the abortion, since abortion after the twelfth week of pregnancy is a significant and more risky procedure for the mother. They will have feelings towards the clergyperson even though they have asked for his or her help. Feelings are very complex towards the clergy because, unlike other helpers, they represent in a special way our ultimate dependence and helplessness. Pastors also have feelings about being asked for help in crisis and about the very mixed expectations that are placed upon them.

Our first response in such a situation can be to evade the feelings. In my experience, this is an unfortunate response, for the result can be an empty, listless examination of moral options. Also, the couple may suffer more depression following their decision than would be the case if given a chance to talk about their feelings. A psychological study of a few such parents showed that serious depression occurred in both parents following abortion for genetic reasons.[1] Good moral counseling begins with an attempt to clear the air and be honest about feelings. Also, our feelings are vital to locate our most deeply *felt* values and beliefs. Moral action in this situation begins with a response to feelings about self and others, including the fetus, and about being in such a situation at all.

Secondly, the couple and counselor will be responding to the *moral* expectations upon them. They face the question, "What ought we to do in this situation? We have a diagnosis of X disease." To move from the feelings *about* self, others, and the situation to the question of *oughtness* is a signal that we respond to sources of moral guidance. It is important in pastoral counseling to make a move from feelings to the ought question, since we want to teach that we should make decisions on appraisals of values or rules that include, but also transcend feelings. At this point, an examination of the alternatives will be needed. Abortion is one choice. The couple can also plan for childbirth, either with the intention of raising the affected child or placing the child for adoption or institutionalization. As the options are examined, the facts and different systems of morality (teleological and deontological) held by individuals will color and shade the way questions are asked and answered. Adequate facts are vital for good moral counseling. The physician would have already informed the couple about the disease in question and any therapy that may exist. If the couple has areas of ignorance that need to be filled in, the decisionmaking needs to be done with the physician. In cases of serious genetic disease for which there is no therapy, my own view is that abortion is morally valid until there is a therapy.

By "serious genetic disease," I mean a disease in which the child struggles for all or the majority of its life simply to survive the disease, without adequate therapy, and that the child's chances for human growth and communication would be completely or to a great degree submerged or overwhelmed by the disease. For example, galactosemia, an inborn inability to utilize sugars found in milk, can be treated successfully with a diet therapy. Cleft palate and lip can be corrected surgically. Both of these can be detected prenatally with amniocentesis or fetoscopy. To me, it would not be morally valid to abort for these conditions, since they are treatable. Other diseases are more complex. Sickle cell disease can be diagnosed prenatally by obtaining fetal blood, but there is no therapy for the disease. Sickle cell disease has a great spectrum of consequences ranging from death, to very few symptoms, to pain. Thousands of individuals have been helped to live with the pain and crises of the disease, but their lives are often dominated by the side effects of pain medication and blood transfusions. Thus there is a "chance" that the child can spend a lifetime of struggle and pain, perhaps ending in death due directly to the disease. With a sex-linked disease like hemophilia or muscular dystrophy, usually the couple can know only the sex of the fetus. Fetoscopy that obtains blood and skin from the fetus for tests is very scarce at present. Without this procedure, one only knows that the odds are 50 percent that the male fetus has the disease. The opposite is also true, so abortion may result in killing a normal male fetus. And the complexities continue.

Response to *moral* action upon us entails responding to conflicting loyalties and values. The issues and values should be identified and explored. The couple will want their decision to be consistent with other decisions they have made; but, since they are in the first generation *ever* making such decisions, they have few precedents. A Catholic father of one affected child who shared with me his view on elective abortion said, "I still *feel* the same way. I was petrified at the thought of having to choose to abort my own child. I would have done it, though, for the sake of saving my family. I am . . . of two minds on the subject—my feelings take me one way and my mind another."[2] He described his feelings as duty-bound (deontological) and his mind as consequentially oriented (teleological). His choice of words is important. Mind is generally preferred over feelings. Actually, he reveals two systems of values that he has assimilated, and in *this* situation (though not in all), he would have made his decision to abort on consequentialist grounds. He made a decision to let the affected fetus be born and to keep and raise his first child, who had Down syndrome, on largely deontological grounds.

This brings me to a third response in the decision about abortion, namely, the response to ethical demands upon us. The differences between *moral* and *ethical* demands are subtle but important to remember. In morality, we are expected to abide by certain rules or norms designed to reduce conflict in contests between individuals, interest groups, and society. "Do not harm," "do not kill," "be fair" are examples. Morality encourages reciprocity and sublimation of the self in the interest of the community. An ethical demand is similar but different. Ethics demands that we restrict self-interest and present our reasons why one or the other alternative in a conflict would be in the "best interests" of the individuals or groups involved in the contest or conflict. To respond to an ethical demand is to give a reasoned argument that spells out the principle(s) involved in following one or another course of action. Also, whenever we propose breaking or changing a rule in the moral code, we are obliged to give our reasons in an ethically defensible manner. We assert that "we are expected" to present ethical arguments but, in reality, many decisions are made publicly and privately without any rational or argued presentation of reasons. In a society that values reason and due process, however, the presentation of arguments is an indispensable element. The counselor can help the couple make this reponse by assuming different roles in the interview. Suppose there is a child at home with the same disease that has been detected in the fetus. Taking the part of the ill child is an effective way of asking for an ethical argument of their reasons. Why is it in the best interest of their child and other children who have the disease to abort the fetus? Why is it in the best interest of all children to do so? And so forth. One can also take the role of a leader in a group devoted to rehabilitation of those affected with the disease in question. The purpose of ethics is to move the people in the conflict from the most self-interested level to a more general level, where they momentarily transcend the conflict and evaluate the options in less heated ways. The couple might justify abortion in terms of the child's "right to be happy and healthy." Where does this "right" come from? Do they really want to argue that way in a society that does not recognize or act on a "right to health?"

Another level of response involves the *beliefs* of the couple and the counselor. They will respond in the light of an interpretation they make of what is happening. The couple's religious beliefs condition the interpretation they make. Some have no stated beliefs that relate to the situation. To them, religion is something to do in church and abortion is something you do when you make a mistake. There is an emptiness and shallowness about the way they approach the problem. Some believe God sent the problem in the form of a defective gene and ask questions about how God can do such a thing to a baby. They see themselves as confronted by a divine power that determines, that kills as well as makes alive. Some see themselves as involved in an impending disaster that can be prevented, and that not to act would be contrary to God's will.

The feelings, moral rules, ethical demands, and beliefs are not separable into neat categories in the actual situation. They are interwoven and dynamically related, making up the various dimensions of a response. To be able to respond to the many dimensions is the beginning of responsibility. To evade most of the dimensions by saying, "We have no choice but to . . ." is, in religious language, to fall into sin, to respond by sidestepping the problem of choice.

II

THREE LETTERS ABOUT
GOD AND GENES

I wrote this material not so much with the hope of reaching a particular person who asked me for religious help, but to straighten out my own attitudes about cries for help and my role as a clergyperson. To the extent that other clergy hear the question of theodicy, "Why did God allow this to happen?" and quake within themselves as I did, these extended second thoughts may be helpful.

The first letter (Chapter 7) reflects on a meeting with a distressed mother following the termination of a pregnancy diagnosed for a serious genetic disorder. The second letter (Chapter 8) represents my study of the question she asked me. The final letter (Chapter 9) reflects on the theme of God's goodness in the context of possible treatment for genetic disorders.

7. A Meeting in Retrospect

Dear Friend,

We first met after your brave attempt to have a healthy child, knowing yourself that you were the carrier of a genetic disorder. On that day, you did more for me than I for you. You asked me a question that took root in my life: "Why does God give so many terrible things to children?"

Now I am the one who needs your help. I should set the record straight about what I did that day. I also need a second chance to respond to you and anyone else who feels punished by God when a child is born with a genetic disorder.

You and I talked in your hospital room after the termination of your pregnancy. You were in great emotional and religious despair but you were very honest and open. You said, "I feel terrible about this, but I don't deserve it. I tried to be a good mother." You really did not need help to reveal your feelings, but these feelings troubled you greatly. You felt defiled and punished. Defilement is an experience of being trampled on, soiled, or contaminated. You also felt punished by God.

As you talked about your religious beliefs, you openly broke into tears and clenched your teeth with rage. You shook your fist at the sky and exclaimed, "Why does God give so many terrible things to children!" You wept with great sobs and continued bitterly, "I prayed to God to give me a healthy baby. But you see what happened? I have lost faith in God!"

My response was to try to persuade you to change your concept of God. As I recall, I said, "You believe God causes and controls everything. That belief causes you a lot of trouble. In your view, every cell moves at God's command. You should distinguish between God and nature, between God and genes." My memory is that you listened politely and stopped weeping so desperately. I used an analogy to shake you loose from what I thought was outworn thinking. I said, "You have children at home who are normal, don't you?" You said that you did. "You keep them in the yard for a few years for protection, but then, eventually, you allow them to venture out and explore the world?" You were quieter and acknowledged that you did these things. "Well," I continued, "would you keep your children penned up indefinitely?" You answered in the negative. Making my point, I said, "God is like a parent who allows us to encounter the risks and freedom of life. You can choose to live in the yard where everything is safe and you are taken care of by a divine parent who controls literally everything, or you can choose to live in a larger world with risks and freedom." I also quoted the Psalmist, "The earth is the Lord's and all that is in it" (Ps. 24:1), to make a point that the earth (genes) is *not* the Lord. I said the Scripture teaches us that God and nature are different. You said that you could see what I was getting at and it made you wonder about your childhood and religion. Shortly after exchanging intentions to keep in touch, I left your room.

In retrospect, when I am honest, I know that I stepped aside from many things that day. Your feelings terrified me with their intensity. I did not say that I felt afraid. I was also angry that you were blaming God for what you knew to be the risks of your decision. I said nothing about anger. Further, you reminded me what I feel about my parents, who were deafened by neonatal disease and accidents, and deprived of the sound of my voice. I get furious when I hear about a God with the power to prevent such things. But I said nothing about my past pain to you.

With these elements, my response to you then was somewhat beside the point. I gave you a lecture on two levels. On one level I said, "God permits these kinds of things to happen in the interest of preserving freedom, which God also created," and on another, I told you in effect not to be honest with me about your experience of

God. I might have asked you to tell God directly in prayer what you felt. I might have helped you, if you needed it, to put your feelings into words. That was my job, but I did not do it because I tried so hard to control myself. I also backed off from you, and I apologize. Now I want to come closer again, alongside you rather than behind a lecture platform.

My response was also unfitting in a second way. If I had been intellectually honest, I would have brought up my disappointment in the argument I gave you that day. The technical name for it is the "free-will defense" of God's power and goodness in the face of evil. Your question, "Why does God give such terrible things to children?" raises the profound theological problem called theodicy, or how we explain that we can trust God even in the midst of evil. The book of Job is perhaps the best example of how suffering people struggle to be sane and loyal to religious traditions after some terrible event.

I was trapped by your question and glib in my answer. I have often been asked to minister to persons affected by the consequences of evil deeds or events. I have often felt defensive and apologetic as I argued that God was all-powerful (omnipotent) and all-good (omnibeneficent) despite the existence of evil. The more I continued to hold these ideas as I had been taught them, the more intellectually dishonest I felt. If I agreed with you that God had *sent* the gene, I would have had to indict God for the evil that had befallen you. From that it would follow that God was responsible for evil in all cases. But I said nothing to you about my own troubled mind. I was dissembling more than a bit when I confidently argued what I doubted with a large part of my mind.

I was not prepared, emotionally or intellectually, to take the risks of meeting you on your own ground. You were ready to do battle with God, and I was not. I was not willing to pursue the logic of your question, that is, "If God creates everything, and if God controls everything, including evolution, and if evolution involves mutations like the one that caused the death and loss of fulfillment for your child, then God must be responsible for evil in this and all cases. If this is true, how can such a God be worthy of worship?

I cannot recover the lost opportunity to have treated myself with as much self-respect as you gave me by your example. I do have a choice now, though, not to continue to act in the same way. I can reflect on what I learned from you and our encounter. Perhaps we can also help others.

I realize now that people who ask for help directly benefit more in the long run than if someone else asks for them or offers unsolicited advice. In general, I like to hear from patients first, rather than from their doctors. I have found that counseling with a patient is much more productive if that person has requested my presence than if he or she has been surprised by a drop-in visit.

When I visited you in your hospital room I might have suggested that the physician be there, too, if you had wanted her to be. I'll bet that she needed to know that you forgave her for not being God-like enough to guarantee you a healthy child. I also bet that she wished that you not hold a grudge against her. I could have made sure about these things. Were you angry at her? Most parents who lose their wished-for child are angry at the doctor. Was I a poor substitute for her?

Perhaps you were angry at your doctor for your bad luck and, rather than tell her, you started in on God. You did have a legitimate cause against God, but are you sure that you were as honest with the doctor as you were with me about God? If not, then I did you no favor to miss the chance to help you to be straightforward.

Suppose that I had been more responsible and you heard from the physician that the minister wanted you to ask him directly to come and see you? How would you have felt? Irritated, outraged? Why doesn't he come right over when he hears about *my* trouble? I would have rather heard that from you than have assumed that under the circumstances you would automatically want to see me. Then I would have known that you could speak for yourself and that you were ready to talk with a minister.

But you were numb. The physician was numb. When I heard about it, I went numb. I acted without testing myself or my feelings. When great trouble comes, not only do our feelings shut down, but our ability to respond creatively to help one another can be paralyzed. What did you feel like when you heard about the diagnosis? Was it not like a knife had cut you in two? I have heard others say "something in me died," when they described the death of those hopes. Is it not like being in a void? Chaos reigns, your world flies apart.

No, I did you no favor to come unbidden. If you recall, I had a chance to correct it by asking you first if you wanted my help. But I simply presumed that you did, much in the way physicians used to presume that patients give their consent to treatment by showing up at the clinic or office. More important, I missed the chance to tell you that the help I had to offer was risky but worth trying in the long run.

What I did was dangerous to everyone, especially to myself. It is dangerous to walk into great trouble numbly, having tested no one or myself. What if you had been suicidal and I blithely walked in? I left you and the physician in the void and chaos you felt by not risking the perfectly obvious thing. Everyone knows that those who ask get more help. Correct? You hear it all your life. So why did I go against conventional wisdom? I was part of the problem by that time, rather than a good companion to you both. When given the choice, a religious leader needs to respond to others in chaos in the belief that life and creativity begin on the other side of chaos. Only the coldness of the void must be scattered.

You had suffered a terrible blow. You were entitled to be numb and withdrawn. But I was not entitled to pretend that I did not know enough to find you had some resources of your own. Otherwise, how shall we really begin the process to find religious help? If you cannot ask me for help, how will you ask God to help you and have it mean anything to you?

Of course, it is possible to give up all together and believe that there is *no* meaning in life. All is unending Chaos, forevermore. I recall being told (I cannot remember the origin) about a scene in a novel. The protagonist is dreaming before a major decision. He dreams that he jumps from an airplane at night, and pulls the rip-cord on the parachute. On the way down, he looks around at all of the other people in the world jumping from planes, floating down through the moonlit sky. He worries about keeping his shrouds out of the way of others and keeping himself from being hit by others on their way down. He thinks to himself that he is doing a pretty good job on the way down. He looks below and sees nothing but blackness. He realizes with a start that there is no bottom, no destination below. In a cold sweat, the dreamer awakes and takes the dream's message into himself. The best we can do in this world is a little justice on the way down to nothing at all. Stay out of others' way and do not let them get in your way. But justice really does not matter in the long run, since there is no point in the journey. The Void is God. You have the choice.

But I was more in a void than you, if I remember my spiritual state. As the young say today, I was "out of it." The ancients called it a state of sin, but they did not mean a moral offense. They meant "missing the point" or "going astray." I missed a lot, not only between you and your physician but between you and your husband. Where was he? Why wasn't he with you when you were suffering so? But again, I said nothing about that to you.

You were not long in a void. You were very much alive. You had feelings, you felt hurt, angry, punished. You were trying to make sense of what had happened to you. My job was to make sure you had cleared the decks of all the anger you owed to the human beings on the scene before you gave God what you felt was due. If you cannot speak directly to others, how can you speak directly to God? I think that we learn to pray authentically this way. You were entitled to feel angry at God, but I used my lecture to blunt your opportunity. You should have swallowed your politeness and told me to listen. You had trusted the power and goodness of God, as you had been taught these ideas, and your trust had been shattered. I have since been with other parents like you, and they felt this way whether they were religious or not. "What did I do to deserve it?" was your question. Every small and large moral lapse you ever had must have rushed into your mind.

Is it not the greatest absurdity when the God you are supposed to trust becomes a punishing enemy? You felt defiled and made to suffer. I tell you that your experience of God links you and me to a shadowy past that lives on within us. A philosopher, Paul Ricoeur, writes that the oldest human memory is dread of a retributive power that takes vengeance on persons who have wronged the order of things. "If you suffer, if you are ill, if you fail, if you die, it is because you have sinned."[1] As a religious leader, I should have stood by you in your experience and not abandoned you, in effect, for the sake of the comfort of my own ideas. I should have seen you through your need to live through the terror of the experience that God is an enemy.

You were entitled to some help to put your feelings towards God into words. Have you read the Psalms? Almost every psalm involves vivid expressions from the human heart to God. The psalmists, poets, and musicians, express every imaginable motive and experience to God. The most memorable Psalms are the ones that embody the experiences of being punished or forsaken by God, and especially the experience of being threatened by death in the presence of God.

I was not a responsible religious leader that day. I did what many clergy do when people express religious needs. I did not ask you what you wanted me to do about it. I took it on myself to give you an answer. I might have asked you if you wanted to pray to God directly, if you believed that God hears prayers. You certainly knew what you felt. You could have done it easily. If you had tried prayer in the past, and you had the courage to try to have a healthy baby against difficult odds, you certainly must have had the courage to speak to God directly about how you felt treated by the Power and Goodness that you once trusted.

If you had felt unable to speak to God directly, you could have told me what you wanted to say, and I could have said it for you. Is that not a role that priests have played for eons? If you had asked me, and if I had helped you to put your feelings towards God into words, I imagine that we would have said together:

O God, I hate you and fear you!
I trusted you and your ways that
I faithfully learned from your priests and people.
You are supposed to be the Creator,
But I suffer from one of your mistakes. Why me
Rather than the woman down the street with four healthy children?
You are supposed to be an all-powerful God.
And you are supposed to be all-good, perfect Love.
Answer me then, Almighty One. If it was within your power
To correct the mistake and you did not,
If you deliberately withheld your power,
Then why should I not hate and fear you?

> You are supposed to love me. How could you love me
> Or my child and not be moved to stop what happened?
> Why should I demean myself by ever again going to
> My knees before the God, distant hand that sends
> Good to one child and evil to another?
> O God of my fathers, I am ashamed of you and your handiwork!
> I long never again to hear of your power and goodness
> For evil has overtaken me and swallowed me up.

If I let myself be in your place, I imagine that you might have felt angry enough to shout, even scream these things. I shall never forget your fist shaking at the sky. Why not put those feelings and that gesture into words? What happens when you do? When I do it, I do not feel as helpless and hopeless, even towards God, whose ways I do not understand. At least, I have some ground on which to stand, if only to speak for myself.

At this point, our work together would have come to a crucial turning point. I see you suffering. You feel that you are being punished. I help you to speak directly to others and to God about your experience. What then? The issue is how committed you are to being punished forever. I should have helped you to find an answer to that question within yourself. Perhaps you would have been shocked again and numbed to find out just how deep was your sense of worthlessness as the bearer of a mutant gene. There is something in all of us that responds to the invitation to be punished forever, but it is sharper in those who feel stigmatized by the world. Those who feel inferior (and who does not feel inferior to someone else?) endlessly torture themselves with feelings of self-hatred and the desire to be destroyed.

Here we are in a crisis where there is nothing in the power of any human being to deliver you from the bottomless despair you feel. You, and only you, know how long you can hate yourself for being who you are and not someone different. Who will help you out of this pit?

Perhaps you would have turned to me and said again, "But why did God do it to *me*, when I tried so hard?" I might have observed that you are acting like you really do not want help with what is troubling you most. How much punishment do you need? Do you want to spend eternity groveling? I can arrange for you to meet some people who can help you with that assignment. They labor day and night in the grip of the final vision of the fires of punishment that inevitably consume every shred of wickedness. There is no escape for them. You can join them.

You have a choice, even in the midst of despair. If you and only you ask God for help with your problem of being bound up with hating who you are, you may discover what others have found who come to this pass. This state is like a "body of death" (Rom. 7:24), where every relationship is dying because of your need to be punished for being the special person you are. You can ask God to love you and accept you, even though you yourself cannot find the power anywhere else to rescue yourself from the pits of self-hatred.

If you ask God for acceptance, you will find it. The teaching of the Lord is firm and true that if we seek, we find; if we knock, it will be opened (Matt. 7:7). But you are the one who has to do the asking. No one else can do it for you. That is simply the way it is.

Venturing out to ask God's help with the unworthiness in ourselves leads to a realization of the love of God that can deliver us, but not permanently, from the self-hatred that endangers us and those who care for us. We can entrust our unworthy selves to God, and experience God's inexhaustible love for us, but the expectation is that we continue to grow after the experience of deliverance. What is more, we can fall back, and do, into the same pattern of living that drove us originally to seek God's help. We continue to need help even after profound change with the need to be punished.

In his small but rich book on the evolution of religion, Alfred North Whitehead made the intriguing observation, never fully developed elsewhere, that "Religion is what the individual does with his own solitariness. It runs through three stages, if it evolves to its final satisfaction. It is the transition from God the void to God the enemy, and from God the enemy to God the companion."[2] My problem as a religious leader with you was that I was too greedy. I wanted to begin with telling you about God the companion without paying the price of being with you at the previous, necessary stages of your experience of God. You gave me an invitation, but I missed the significance of it. Clergy do have this problem, you know, they want to *teach,* but we do it more often when the ground is not prepared. Then we wonder why no one listens. If I had it to do over again, I would have saved all of my teaching until just this point. Then we would have been able to pursue the question of "why" after having cleared the air about just who was punishing who and why. As long as your spiritual emptiness and infinite capacity for self-punishment remain the issues, all of the scientific and religious teaching in the world will not meet your needs.

I say this as much to myself as to other clergy, because it is so crucial to our work. When clergy respond to cries for help from those who have been injured by the terrors of life and death, we are called to work first in the icy void of spiritual emptiness and the fires of self-punishment. Only when some kind of resolution comes should we take steps to encourage the formerly helpless one to seek help from science and better theological arguments. The role of the clergy is to be faithful companions in the religious process, not to substitute for scientists or professional theologians. Our task is to send people to the help of medicine and theology with their anxiety and despair in a state of transformation rather than being primary obstacles to the education that can follow.

Genetic counselors can spend hours explaining the origin of a mutation and its risks, but the information does not penetrate beneath the core of the desire to punish oneself mercilessly for being a carrier. Sophisticated theological arguments *about* God's power and goodness do not *in themselves* have the power to deliver suffering people from despair and lead to belief *in* God, in the sense of trusting in God. Nothing else can replace the need of the individual to ask sincerely for God's help, and that is the role of faithful companions: to test the sincerity of that deepest cry for help with burdens of life that threaten to undo us.

8. Why Did It Happen? Why Didn't God Prevent It?

I have done some research on these questions, and I offer it to you for what it is worth. Two assumptions are behind the research. If you simply want to read what follows, you need not share these assumptions. But if you want my help with the question you originally asked, "Why does God give so many terrible things to children?" you do need to share these assumptions.

First, an enlightened religious view *should not* be held apart from science. A sincere religious outlook welcomes all ways of knowing and is afraid of none. We are taught by Jesus (Mark 12:29b) to love God with all the mind, as well as the heart, soul, and strength. We can arrive at the best answer to "why?" by first considering the best scientific evidence. Rather than seeking God in the gaps of what we do not know, why not seek at first God's ways in and behind what we do know?

The second assumption is that if obstacles to belief in God exist in the form of defective arguments that leave us frustrated and in a dilemma, we ought to try to remove them by better arguments. Theological arguments that try to make sense of God's ways are not the same as God's ways. We have latitude to reject a mode of argument, especially if it defeats the goal of the religious process to restore trust in the goodness of living even in the face of evil. Let me give you a preview of the argument here that I ask you to consider. Although it is true that God cannot prevent the possibility of evil done by mutant genes, since not even God can determine the being of another, God does set the optimal limits to freedom for all creatures, from the most ancient particle to the newest recombinant gene made by scientists, in such a way that more good than evil is possible. I hope to persuade you in the end that we can worship God without reservation about his power and goodness *and* strive to find basic therapies for genetic disorders, without denial that evil is real and genuine. For the rest of this letter I think it will help if I get more specific and focus on one of the genetic disorders that physicians encounter. For this particular dicussion I will take Lesch-Nyhan syndrome as an example. However, the same principle of explanation could apply to other disorders such as Duchenne's muscular dystrophy and hemophilia.

Physicians now know that Lesch-Nyhan syndrome is caused by a deficiency on the genetic level. Purine biosynthesis is central to the function of normal cells; without purines there is no life. A purine is a crystalline base that is the parent of compounds of the uric-acid group. In a child with this disorder, an enzyme required in the regulation of purine biosynthesis is deficient. This enzyme is hypoxanthine-guanine phosphoribosyl-transferase, a forbiddingly long name. Scientists call it HGPRT for short. In plain language, one or more mutant genes copy an inaccurate message in the making of HGPRT that results in uric acid poisoning of the child. Patients excrete three to six times more uric acid than normal individuals. Every HGPRT message in every cell in their bodies is faithfully copied from an original misprint.

Let us review what is known about the evolution and transmission of Lesch-Nyhan syndrome. Lesch-Nyhan syndrome is named for the two physicians who first identified it in young male patients in 1964. Physicians believe that the syndrome is a more destructive first cousin to gout, or clinical gouty arthritis, a painful metabolic disease that inflames the joints due to excessive deposits of salts of uric acid. It is also known that animals below the higher primates (apes) have an enzyme in the liver, uricase, that breaks down uric acid to such an extent that no animal below apes on the evolutionary ladder have gout. Dogs and cats, for instance, do not suffer from uric acid disorders. At some point in the evolution of higher pri-

mates, however, uricase disappeared from the picture. One mutation, probably in a series of mutations, made Lesch-Nyhan syndrome possible.

At another point in evolution, however, more relevant to humans, the gene(s) that encode for HGPRT located on the X-
chromosome. To understand the significance of this location, I
want to teach you, if you do not know it, the analogy of the gene
library.

Our bodies are organized by billions of cells. Richard Dawkins, a
British zoologist, coined the analogy to the human body of a gigantic library containing as many rooms as there are cells.[2] Each cell is
one room. In each room there is a bookcase, the nucleus of the cell.
In each bookcase are the plans for the whole building. The plans are
printed in forty-six matched volumes (chromosomes). The genes are
analogous to pages in the volumes. Genes are composed of DNA
molecules that can be likened to printed words on the page, or the
details of the plan. You must have seen pictures of the helix-shaped
chains of DNA molecules that are the building blocks of the genes.

The alphabet used to compose the messages of DNA are combinations of four nucleic acids that always pair with their opposites.
These four building block letters are adenine, thymine, cytosine,
and guanine (heard of the last one?), but simply shortened to A, T,
C, and G. These four nucleotides comprise two groups of molecules, the purines (A and G) and the pyramidines (T and C). A
deficiency in HGPRT is a mistake on the page that instructs for
HGPRT, needed to make purine synthesize correctly in every room
in the library. If the instructions are incorrect in one room, they
will be incorrect in every room.

To learn how this inborn error happened, we must cover some
ground about biological evolution. Ernst Mayr, professor emeritus
of zoology at Harvard University, explains that evolution by natural
selection is a two-step process.[2] The first step is the production of
diversity, a literal explosion of differences found in hundreds of
thousands of species of insects, plants, and animals. Every biological individual is different. Just as no two fingerprints are alike,
every sperm and egg is unique.

What causes this immense diversity? Probably the greatest cause
of variety is from the event of recombination or "crossing over" that

occurs during the making of the sex cells, the sperm and the egg. Do you recall that these cells contain only twenty-three chromosomes, one half of forty-six? A nice invention, without which reproduction could not take place! You will also recall that the chromosomes that composed your egg from which your children were conceived were prepared in the testes and ovary of your own parents. These organs perform a totally different function—when it comes to cells—than any others. They reduce cells with forty-six chromosomes to twenty-three and store them for future use. *Meiosis* is derived from the Greek word for reduction. Meiotic divisions happen when cells with forty-six chromosomes divide to form sex cells with twenty-three chromosomes.

The genetic composition of each sperm and egg is different because, during the making of a sperm or egg, pieces of each chromosome from the father change places with the exactly matching pieces of chromosomes from the mother. If you remember the concept of "matched volumes," then imagine pages of the volumes in loose-leaf binders. During meiosis, pages from one volume swap with those from the matching volume. The result is a complete sex cell library composed of equal bits of forty-six volumes but now comprising twenty-three volumes. The complete forty-six volume library happens at reproduction. The "scrambling" effect of recombination during meiosis promotes variety within and between species. It is also the main reason that children within a family are distinctly different.

The second cause of variety in nature is mutations. Mutations are changes in the genetic material that are inheritable. Mutations can occur at any point on the stair-steps of the double helix. These events involve changes in the sequencing of DNA molecules (in our analogy, the order of words on the page). Without mutation, there would be no evolution, but mutations in themselves do not cause evolution. Do they occur for a reason, such as a master plan for all of the libraries? No, apparently mutations occur at random. At random means that a definite plan is lacking, but there is a probability that mutations occur with a certain frequency. All mutations begin as changes in the messages of DNA molecules. Whether the mutations are harmful or beneficial, in the long run, is a complex problem. Francisco Ayala, professor of genetics at the University of

California, believes that most mutations are harmful since a population is usually well-adapted to its environment. He writes, "Major changes are usually maladaptive, just as a large random change in the construction of a clock (removing a spring or adding a gear) is not likely to improve its functioning."[3]

The third cause of variation is chance events, such as changes in climate, solar conditions, or catastrophes. Some scientists think that dinosaurs disappeared suddenly because of widespread earthquakes. Dr. Mayr points out that most of the variation produced by these three causes (that amount to the first step in evolution) is random, "in that it is not caused by, and is unrelated to, the current needs of the organism or the nature of its environment."[4]

It is not yet known why the particular series of mutations occurred that led the messages for HGPRT to locate on the human X-chromosome, but we do know by experiments in gene mapping that the location is the sex chromosome. I will use the gene library analogy to explain just what "happened."

The forty-six volumes consist of twenty-three pairs of matched volumes. Imagine these numbered as Volume 1a and 1b, and so forth down to 23a and 23b. All of these marked "a" came from the father and "b" from the mother. Each page of every matched pair is about a different subject (e.g., eye color, brain cells, liver cells). Let us say the HGPRT instructions are printed on page six. The genetic instructions for HGPRT, however, are not matched when it comes to males and females. Females have matched pairs of Volume 23, understood as Volume 23a and 23b, since they have two X-chromosomes. The male, however, has twenty-two matched volumes and one pair of unmatched volumes at the twenty-third location. One member of this nonidentical pair, Volume 23b (called X), is just like one of the corresponding female pair and contains the instructions on page six for making HGPRT. The male partner of X, Volume 23a, called Y, does not appear in the female bookcase.

In the library of the female carrier, Volumes 23a and 23b have exactly the same subjects on page six, the making of HGPRT. In Volume 23a, the instructions are correct and in Volume 23b they are incorrect. The first volume was prepared in the testis of her father and the second in the ovary of her mother. In her, the correct message cancels out any harm that might be done by the incorrect message.

In the male library, however, the situation is different. In each conception of a male who will have Lesch-Nyhan syndrome, he inherits Volume 23b from his mother, whose page six contains the faulty message. His Volume 23b is a Y-chromosome from his father, whose page six does not contain any instructions for HGPRT. So, the faulty message prevails. Fifty percent of the time, his brother inherits Volume 23a from the mother, which contains the correct messages for HGPRT.

Mayr points out that the second step of evolution is the ordering of genetic variety by natural selection.[5] Natural selection is change and adaptation. Change refers to which genotypes (the genetic constitution of an individual) live or die out. Apparently, the survival rates in evolution occur by chance. Adaption refers to the fact that in the great variety of unique individuals, some will have genes that are better suited to the problems and pressures of the environment at the time. We should probably guard against imputing a will, purpose, or foresight to natural selection. If there is such a thing as evolutionary progress, we are the only creatures who can know it. It is certainly unclear what possible advantages the omission of HGPRT instructions from genes might have had, if any, at the time that this mutation originally appeared.

Natural selection is a cumulative process that ensures that some genetic libraries last longer than others. To thrive genetically, you must be able to leave descendents, and to do this, you must be able to survive until reproduction, or to the age of "fitness." Any condition that increases mortality in youth will decrease fertility. Any condition that decreases fertility will also reduce the chances of those genes being able to survive. Natural selection is a process that determines which species last and which do not. Almost all of the young males with Lesch-Nyhan die in their teens and do not reproduce themselves.

In addition to longevity and fertility, the environment is a third vital factor in natural selection. When the environment changes slowly or radically, pressures build up to select against the reproduction of certain genotypes and affected individuals. The basic message of natural selection is that all life evolves by the different rates of survival of creatures that reproduce themselves.

How does Lesch-Nyhan disease survive, since none of the affected boys has ever been known to reproduce? Since all the affected individuals die, one-third of the total affected genes for Lesch-Nyhan syndrome are lost. New examples of the disease are reported with a frequency that indicates that there are fresh mutations on the X-chromosomes of girls and a few boys in each generation that lead to the disease.[6]

Why Didn't God Prevent It?

Looking back now to a letter I might write, I could end my letter here and say, "Well, you may not like it, but science is all that is reliable. Anything else will just be speculation and is unknowable anyway, especially if you want to know what God has to do with it." That is an *agnostic* answer to your question. Or, I could go a step further and say, "Your hunch was right, and you should be honest, logical, and stick with it. If God is all-powerful, God could prevent evil. Moreover, if God were all-good, he would want to prevent evil. There is evil, for we have seen the results of genetic disorder. Therefore, God does not exist, at least the all-good, all-powerful God that traditional theists worship." That is an *atheistic* answer.

But I am not willing to sign off here. After studying the question you asked and the ways of answering it, I believe there is a better way than agnosticism, atheism, or the intolerable dilemma of traditional theism. Let me explore the dilemma first, with the help of theologian Schubert Ogden.[7] He points out that the problem is actually a "trilemma," because it is composed of the incompatibility of three assertions: that God is all-powerful, that he is all-good, and that evil is real. Although any two of these assertions can be accepted consistently with another, the addition of the third involves the human mind in self-contradiction. Let me demonstrate.

First, if God is all-powerful, it is within his power to correct the mutant gene that produces such suffering and death. If God is all-good, he will certainly be moved to compassion by such innocent suffering. If God could correct the defect and does not by withholding his power, then God is not good. Therefore an all-good God cannot exist.

Second, if God is all-good, surely he will be moved to compassion by such innocent suffering. If God is affected, moved, or limited by any temporal condition, God is less than absolute in his power. If God can be moved, he is less than absolute in his power and not truly God. Therefore an all-powerful God cannot exist.

Third, if God is all-powerful, he has the power to prevent evil. If God is all-good, he has the compassion to prevent evil. If evil is real, then an all-good, all-powerful God does not exist. Therefore evil is not real.

Most traditional theists attempt to deal with the problem in either one of two ways. First, some say that the act or event is apparently evil when you first see it but turns out to be good by serving a hidden purpose. When evil is viewed from the vantage point of the whole, rather than the part, evil can, in their view, turn out to be good. Eighteenth-century poet Alexander Pope put the idea this way:

> All discord, harmony not understood;
> All partial evil, universal good;
> And, spite of pride, in erring reason's spite,
> One truth is clear, whatever is, is right.[8]

On the strength of this view, you would need to believe that the HGPRT defect was evil *prima facie*, or at first sight, but in the long run was part of a pattern of greater good to be accomplished by God.

The second way is the argument I tried on you originally. The essence of the "free-will defense" of God's power and goodness is that, just as evil can exist because we are free to choose evil, there is such freedom at other levels of life, such as the genetic level. There exists the freedom for mutations to occur. God permits a world in which evil is possible in the interest of preserving freedom, which God also created. The problem with this way of understanding evil is that there is no deliverance from the dilemma we have already reviewed. If God created freedom, then God is finally responsible for evil, since God created the very foundation by which we can choose evil. On the other hand, if we creatures, including the genes, can contradict God's plan by free will (or its equivalent on the genetic level), then this is certainly a challenge to, if not a contradiction of, God's power. God must be in control to be God, and God must have all the power there is. There is a third way, namely, to deny that evil is real.

After what you have been through, would you deny that evil is real? Would those who had lived through Buchenwald and Dachau deny that evil is real? Not and keep their sanity, in my view.

Ways of Thinking About God's Power

Let's examine the way that you and I have imagined God's power or, to use the theological word, God's omnipotence. I assume that we are similar in our intellectual upbringing, because when I examine myself closely on the subject, I too have held the idea that God has a monopoly on power, *if he wanted to use it.* God's power, my thought goes, must be *all* the power there is. In terms of the actual world, this means that God has the power to control events. He could have converted Hitler from his hatred of the Jews. He has the power to prevent mutations that harm and to cause mutations that help. There is no question about the extent of his power! I was taught that God, by definition, is Absolute and in absolute control. Does this sound familiar? There is no escape from the dilemma of this conclusion. God is indictable for evil. At this point, theologians who hold to the "free-will defense" usually resort to the language of mystery. I am unwilling to accept this end-point any longer, because it resolves nothing. In fact, I think it is better to be agnostic than to resort to the language of mystery, better in the sense that at least you do not contribute to a climate where great evils are allowed to go unchallenged because somehow you suppose that God, by withholding his power, allows the evil to happen for a greater purpose.

What is the nature of this traditional thinking that jumps out to help us absorb some terrible event? In our society, even those who are "secularists" in the sense that they openly disagree with traditional religious teaching about the final meaning of human life are still strongly influenced by a tradition of thinking that has been called the *philosophia perennis,* or Christian philosophy. The heart of this philosophy is that God is the Absolute and that everything that has existence is absolutely dependent upon God. Only God is truly free, that is, not created by any other power that can rival his power. The heart of traditional theism teaches us to understand what it means for anything to count as actual and real (my translation of the word "metaphysics") is in its relationship to God. God alone is understood as self-creative, truly undetermined by anything else, totally determined from within himself. On this understanding, God can do everything that is not logically self-contradictory. God cannot make a circle square, but God can certainly make a circle and a square. Thus God's absoluteness is the source of all reality. To accept this absoluteness and conform to it is the proper role of every creature. God has all of the power there is, and every event is controlled or controllable by God.

An alternative to this kind of thinking is process thinking. Remember that at the level of metaphysics human thought tries to distill the most fundamental principles of what it means to be anything at all. I call this activity our "master interpretations" of reality. In process thinking, for something to count as *actual*—and this means existing in fact or reality—"is to be an instance of process, or creative synthesis, and therefore, a free response to the free decisions of others already made."[9] What does this mean? Think of the meaning of what you are now doing as you read this page. You respond, no doubt, in agreement or disagreement, to my choice to write to you. You also respond to many others in your past who have influenced your thinking. Your parents are there, your teachers, perhaps one very influential person. You, in effect, create yourself now by responding to me and to them. All of those in your past were self-creative in that they also responded to many others in their own freedom. They were free to shape you. You are who you are because of these many contributors to your history. But (and this is an important *but)* you are free to differ with their views and with mine about the subjects on this page. You have the power of self-determination. You, and you alone, bring yourself to these choices.

At least two steps are involved in creative synthesis. First, anything actual freely creates itself in the present by responding to the past responses of others. These others are also self-created and have contributed their pasts to the new moment. You, and every other actual thing, are a center of this creative synthesis with the past and present. But there is a second step, a movement toward the future, in which you bring forth something new. You will take your response to me and to others in your past into your future. You will contribute yourself to others, your children, and others you have not yet met, and you will freely respond to them. You will help to create others by your future responses. You have the power to help determine others. To complete the statement about the process view, "self-creation" is the key understanding of what it means for anything to be at all. You and every other existing entity are centers of a creative synthesis of past, present, and future.

We know now that even genes participate, to a certain degree, in such a creative synthesis. A gene, or a group of genes, responds not only to the information programmed in the genes that were its direct predecessors, but also to signals that come from the environment. As genes replicate themselves, they respond to the action upon them of the past and the present. Genes also penetrate forward into the future by replication and mutation. In every new replication of genes in the present and future, somewhat novel and unique results can be expected. Just as you cannot be determined completely by your past, so it is even with a gene, although the degree of freedom you have is much greater in every way than the case of a gene. Remember the analogy of the many-roomed library —every nucleus of every cell likened to a bookcase containing the architect's plans for the whole building? Well, the contents of every bookcase, even in the same building, are slightly different. Why? Because a brain cell is not a liver cell, and so forth. And a brain cell tomorrow and the next day will not be exactly the same in every feature, just as you and I are not the same in every feature, each successive day that we live and renew our experience. The principle here is that nothing whatever, including God, has the power to determine completely the being of something else. Everything that is, from cellular to human life, from the simplest to the most complex, has its own degree of freedom.

We should conclude that not even God, who has the greatest imaginable power, has all of the power there is, since everything is to this extent self-creative. In the language of metaphysics, self-creation is the first principle. We must then reformulate the idea of

God's all-powerfulness or omnipotence to mean all of the power that God can be imagined to have, consistent with there being other things in the universe having the kind of effective, self-determining power that is required by their capacities. A brain cell has enough self-determining power to be a brain cell and to do what it should do. And, to go back to our earlier example, the genes that code for HGPRT, or any other genetic disorder, have enough self-determining power to do their task.

While we are at it, let's look at the meaning of God's power another way. What does it mean to *have* power? Ogden points to the fact that to have power always means to have it in relation to something else.[10] In short, having power is a *social* reality. Having power means to be able to influence or control the choices of others, as well as one's own choices. You and I have power with our children, because we can influence or control their choices. But my power or your power is certainly not all the power there is in the family. There is a second meaning of power, namely, power is divided. Children have power, certainly less than mine or yours, but nonetheless real. They have the power to be affected by our influence, and their power affects us. This "two-way street" is at the heart of what it means to have power, if the word "power" is to refer to anything actual. Power means not only to influence the decisions of others, but to be affected by the decisions of others. Everything that is has some power, however small, of self-determination and reciprocity, including the gene(s) for HGPRT.

So, by definition, God does not have a monopoly on power in relation to genes or anything else that is actual in the world. Since everything that is actual has two kinds of power—self-determination, and some power to influence others—God cannot totally determine any event or individual. The gene(s) for HGPRT, for instance, have, in part, been determined by action upon them by other genes and environments, and these genes also have a certain degree of self-determination in relation to present and future. Indeed, the mutation appears afresh today in men and women.

But does not this process idea of omnipotence reduce God's power and make him imperfect rather than perfect? Theologian David Griffin[11] helped me with this question. If it is impossible for God, or any other individual, to completely determine the being of another actual individual, then the concept of God as the Absolute Controller of events is "verbalizable" but "not coherently conceivable." You can say it out loud, "God controls genes," but you cannot think it without contradicting the evidence of ordinary experience. Have you ever experienced anything that was totally without power of its own? Surely a gene has power. Your own life story attests to it. And what is more ordinary than a gene? The point is that since it is impossible for God, in principle, to be the Absolute Controller of events—the One who sends good genes to some infants and bad genes to others—except in some ideal rather than actual world, there is no limitation on God's perfection if God cannot determine the being of another, including a gene. God confronts the actual world—as it is—in every new moment of creation. God is the power that holds this actual world together. God's power is still the greatest possible power within the many powers that also exist. There is no rational reason, therefore, to believe that God is not perfect. There may be, as Griffin shows, an emotional attachment to an older concept of perfection that is based on God as the Absolute. But such an attachment can be changed gradually over many years and given up for something finer, more in keeping with actuality. What could be more perfect, in the sense of *wholeness*, than a God with the power partly to determine each being that is in the world by setting the limits to each part and particle in such a way as to encourage optimal freedom of all? What could be more perfect, in the sense of inspiring awe and respect, than a God who can hold the universe together in one society without undermining the freedom of each part? Such a God is worthy of worship, from my point of view; and, furthermore, God is worthy of the worship of free creatures.

The result of this argument, in my view, breaks open the heart of the dilemma of the traditional "free-will defense" of God's power and goodness. God is not indictable for events that involve evil, because evil is the result of decisions and outcomes for which God cannot be considered responsible, given a measure of self-determination and influence on the part of each creature. One being (God) cannot guarantee that all of the other beings will avoid evil, just as one being, even a being with perfect power, cannot totally determine the being of others. So, the possibility of evil is as much a part of the actual world as the self-creation of each individual. Why doesn't this possibility of evil defeat the power of God? Griffin makes sense to me when he says that there is a difference between holding the idea that genuine evil is *necessary* (in the sense of inevitable), and holding the idea that the *possibility* of genuine evil is necessary.[12] After all, it is possible that the very best set of circumstances in a situation will be attained. It is not inevitable that evil always accompany the good that can be done. But it is inevitable that the possibility of evil will always be present. So, no being, not even a God with perfect power, can preclude the possibility of evil in an actual, rather than ideal, world. A world without genuine evil is imaginable, and we should hold that such a world is within the realm of possibility. But a world without the possibility of evil is not imaginable, if we are to continue to imagine an actual world with beings who have the power to determine themselves and influence others. God's intent is surely to prevent genuine evil, including the evil done by mutant genes; but not even an omnipotent God can guarantee a world without the possibility of the evil that can be done by genes or any other creature acting in the power of its own self-creation. Therefore God cannot be held responsible for evil in the sense of being responsible for the results of decisions or events such as mutations of genes.

9. God's Goodness and the Future of Genetic Disorders

What about the other side of the problem of theodicy? How can God be truly good in the face of evil? There was an element of moral outrage in your response that day we spoke. Not only had your trust in the arrangements by which God is supposed to be all-powerful been shattered, but your assumption that God is good, compassionate, and loving was in ashes.

You and I were taught the traditional concept of God's goodness. The ideas has four parts. First, God can will only good and not evil. He has no intention to harm any being in the universe. Second, God is perfect. He does not need anything to complete a need or lack. God is empty of any self-interest or desire to "better himself," since God is perfectly good already. And then there were the final two teachings, that God is immutable and impassible. The first term means that nothing in God changes. To change is a sign of imperfection. Everything in time is "perishing" or passing away, and God is *above* time, in the eternal realm. The second term, impassible, means that God is incapable of experiencing pain or suffering. If God is passable, God can be touched. If God can be touched, he can be changed from one state of affairs to another. If God is subject to any control from the outside, God is less than perfect. Is that the concept you were taught? Do you know the hymn that begins, "O God our help in ages past, our hope for years to come"? I wonder how God can be a help if God is so *beyond* the suffering and pain of the world's creatures as to not be affected by the good or the evil of life. What am I doing here in church, I would ask myself, acting as if God could "hear" prayers and yet stuck with a concept that tells me that even if God can hear them, God will not be moved?

When confronted by your question, I was left with a hopeless contradiction. I could not explain how a Goodness conceived along the lines above would not be less than perfectly good if genuinely affected by the pain and suffering you felt because of mutant genes. Not only your question confounded me, but also, how can I square this idea of God's goodness with the portrayal of God's responses in the Bible? God loves, gets angry, yearns for freedom for dispossesed sons and daughters, sends rain on the just and unjust alike, forgives sins, judges the nations, and so forth. The answer is that I cannot hold these two contradictory ideas without mental agony that ends in an understandable moral outrage.

How can we better understand the goodness of God? If you can accept the argument that God's power partly determines each being in the world, but is not all the power there is, then we can take a new step towards a better understanding. Again, following Schubert Ogden's lead, given what has been argued about God's power, you could hold with no contradiction that God's aim in relationship with all other beings, rather than an intent to determine totally their decision, is by God's own free choice "to optimize the limits of all of theirs."[1]

To optimize means to make as perfect, effective, or functional as possible. In effect, God's abiding intent, in relation to every part and to the whole, is to create the best possible world. But God confronts the same actual world that we do in the fullness of the good and evil that actually exists. God's own unique work as Creator, that no other can do, is to hold together the cosmic order that structures our world. Further, God alone presents each creature in each moment with that cosmic order. The point is that God freely chooses to present the limits to every activity in the cosmos in an optimal way, meaning that the limits are set in a way that favors the possibilities of the greatest good and the least possible evil. If the limits were set other than they are, the risk of more evil to opportunity for good would be higher. Does that make sense to you? Perhaps an example would help.

Think of approaching a difficult decision or task. You have the responsibility to give another person critical observations or facts that will likely hurt. I am reminded of my responsibility in visiting you. My responsibility was to help you mature and gain more compassion by your suffering and to oppose the possibility that you might forever act like you were a "special case" that God had singled out for punishment. Another scenario is when a physician is obliged to convey bad news. You can make decisions about the task in an optimal way and ensure that the most good can result. Or you can make decisions less than optimally, and leave it to chance that more evil might result than would be the case if you *tested the limits* of the situation to discover what is possible. I could have done more to test your limits for more discovery about what had happened to you, your family, and your physician. You were capable of so much more than I gave you credit for that day, and so was I. In a similar vein, I have occasionally seen physicians who want to sedate a patient before telling them terrible news or before obtaining consent when the patient is very disturbed.

The right intention for such an encounter is to enter it with all bases covered, including a good impression of what you might do when the facts hurt. Every effort should be made to optimize the good that can be done, without "tinkering" or manipulating the situation to make it easier for you to do the task. If, in spite of efforts to prevent pain without subterfuge, some pain is suffered by the other, there is no way you could have responsibly prevented it, other than to have shifted your responsibility in the first place. I am not simply equating pain and evil, but using the pain that follows disclosure as an example. The possibility of evil is there, but it is not necessary or inevitable that any evil will result.

The optimality of our relationship is plain in how many good possibilities were available in its beginnings. The point is that the possibilities for good always outweigh the possibilities for evil because of the work of God the Creator. Good is not done in the actual situation, however, without a struggle, because the possibility of evil is always there.

Goodness has at least two baselines. To be good means to have the best aim or intent. To be good also means to be responsible in the sense of being affected by the struggle to maximize good and minimize evil. You can set the highest aim for an encounter to be truthful to another, but then allow the situation to deteriorate because you are unresponsive and closed in the actual situation. God's goodness is unsurpassable in this second sense as well. Everything that happens in the struggle of freedom affects God. God is unsurpassed in freely chosen responsibility to and for the struggle to maximize good and minimize evil. God's responsibility is demonstrated in the sense that he opens himself to the living struggle of each and all in their decisions in such a way that each makes a difference to him and he makes a difference to each. How do we know this? In two ways: you can hear from others who experience God's mercy even in the most dire circumstances. The traditions of Israel, the witness of the prophets, especially Second Isaiah and Jeremiah, and the impact of the life and death of Jesus of Nazareth are the most trustworthy sources of the experience of others. Secondly, you can discover for yourself that you walked through "the valley of the shadow of death" with the help of a power that did not abandon you when everything else collapsed. If you ever feel that you make a difference to God, then no one has the power or authority to take that recognition away from you. It can be ignored, but it cannot be denied. If God would not abandon you in your struggle, why would God abandon any other being?

In just this way, we can conceive of God as the Creator with the power to determine partially the free decisions of all others and as the Redeemer to whom the struggles of each and all in freedom makes an ultimate difference. The Creator's abiding aim is to create the best possible world. The Redeemer's abiding aim is to open himself to each and all of the creatures in their struggle to be and remain free within the optimal limits of freedom. I believe that it is in these two affirmations that we make sense of the claim that God *loves* the world. The remainder of my letter takes up the theme of God's goodness in the context of evolutionary development and the search for treatment of genetic disorders.

God's Goodness and Evolution

Let me take you back to something Dawkins, the zoologist, wrote.[2] He said that "of course" there is *no architect* (euphemism for Creator) of the plans in the libraries of all of the cells in the world. Dawkins reminds us that, prior to the last century, the harmonies of the living forms in the world were taken as evidence of the existence of a Master Designer (God) with a plan for everything. After Darwin, some biologists and theologians continued to argue that there was a "drive towards perfection" that controlled evolution. There had to be a final program and a Programmer. This philosophy was known variously as teleology (from the Greek work *telos*, meaning end or purpose), finalism, or vitalism. Dr. Mayr points out that there is no scientific basis for finalism, and that the evidence of biological research shows the unevenness and discontinuity of evolution as well as its continuities.[3] The only constant in biological evolution is the gene, and genes only change by mutation. As we have seen, mutations occur randomly or by chance. Natural selection, selection by survival, does not occur by chance but by adaptation. Mayr cites the work of Simpson to show that, in the evolution of a particular characteristic like larger body size or longer teeth, the evolutionary trend is not consistent. It changes direction and occasionally reverses itself. The most powerful argument against finalism is that so many species become extinct.

If biological evolution does not have an architect, then what is the best understanding of it? Stephen Jay Gould, a paleontologist (one who studies fossils to interpret the life of past geological periods), has written some lucid essays on the meaning of evolution.[4] In one of these, he discusses the choice between metaphors for understanding evolution: a "ladder" or a "bush."[5] Most popular thinking pictures evolution as a ladder. We look for a continuous, unbroken sequence of changes linking a "higher" form of life, such as *homo sapiens*, to a series of "lower" rungs, namely our apelike ancestors and their primate forebears. The ladder image probably stems more from our need to think that we humans are the special, preordained, goal of biological evolution.

Gould says that the fossil record suggests that evolution is like the splitting of the branches of a bush from the larger trunk of parental stock. He shows that there were at least three different but co-existing hominid-like ancestors of humans in Africa between two and three million years ago. His message is that major change in evolution does not occur in slow, gradual changes in large populations, but in faster changes *at the edges* or periphery of larger populations. These faster changes are accomplished in smaller groups that become isolated from the larger group. In these "rapid bursts of speciation," according to Gould, evolution is mainly concentrated, rather than in the step-by-step progress of a species "advancing" up a ladder.

Biologist Theodosius Dobzhansky also refers in his writings[6] to the same phenomenon as "branching," "emergence," or "transcendence." The term "transcendence" could be misunderstood if it were connected to a notion of inevitable progress, as suggested by the ladder metaphor. Let me remind you and myself that natural selection guides the course of evolutionary change. To quote Gould, the essence of Darwinism is that "natural selection is the major creative force of evolutionary change."[7] Natural selection creates the fit, meaning the selection of those variations (genetic changes) that will survive and adapt better in the *local* environment in which those changes are produced. There is no guarantee of moral progress given in and through evolution alone. Principles of perfection that are first cousins to religious ideas of the perfection of God are not to be found controlling evolution. Human beings are responsible for the quality of morality in any time or place.

It is easy to see why evolutionary thinking offends us if we hold a concept of God's power as all the power there is and the companion idea of God's being unaffected by anything that is actual. But once these concepts are reformulated successfully, without reducing in any way the insurpassability of God, there is no necessity to believe that God completely determines biological evolution. God does not totally determine the processes of evolution, whether they be atomic, chemical, or biological. God is the creative order upon which evolution draws in order to be at all, but all types of evolutionary processes function with appropriate freedom within the creative order. There is no good reason, from any standpoint, to hold that God determines evolution.

But there is not a good reason, from a religious standpoint, to hold that God makes no difference at all to evolution. If God makes no difference at all to evolution, then God makes no difference at all to any experience of good or evil. If these experiences occur in any actual world, they occur in a world that is evolving. Between the extreme of claiming that God totally determines evolution as its architect and the extreme of saying that God makes no difference at all in the observable, evolving world, there is another possibility. Namely, God sets the limits for evolution in an optimal way and is affected by every experience of good and evil in the context of evolution.

Think with me a moment about the meaning of the terms good and evil. We are used to thinking of good as the prevention of harm and evil as doing harm. This definition of these terms is commonplace. But good and evil are richer, more complex ideas. David Griffin[8] points out two criteria of intrinsic goodness that contrast to intrinsic evil, or evil that is destructive by its very nature. If anything is good, it has the marks of harmony and intensity. Let me illustrate these criteria with an example.

I don't know about you, but I am happiest at the end of a day full of a rich variety of experiences, and when I have made a good stab at my own part in them. I come home in awe at how much more there is to be learned. I am apt to say, "Now, that was a good day." The days that are bad and most miserable involve one of two things. Either the conflict has been so great as to prevent resolution of any differences, or the opposite, absolutely nothing happened. On the one hand, there can be intolerable conflict of the kind that overwhelms differences and makes no allowance for variety. We call this experience discord. On the other hand, there can be boredom, monotony, or as Griffin puts it, "unnecessary triviality."[9] We are much more likely to notice the first kind of evil because suffering and harm result.

The second kind of evil is not so obvious, but just as much loss results. These losses follow from the lack of intensity, or from minimizing differences and variety. We can see these losses vividly in the process of evolution but it is harder for us to see them in our own personal or social lives. For example, if a species does not have enough genetic variety to enable it to adapt to changing circumstances, it will become extinct. Richard Lewontin[10] gives an example of plants in a region that becomes drier because of changes in rainfall. Plants can respond by evolving deeper roots or a thicker cuticle on the leaves, but only if their available genes (that is, the gene pool) contain enough variety for longer roots and thicker leaves. Indeed, there must be enough variety so that the plant species can change as fast as the environment changes. If the variety is lacking, the species will die. One of the great evils loose in the world today is wanton destruction of biological species by pollution and the degradation of forests and streams. A respected study of the global problem of loss of plant and animal genetic resources suggests that between 15 and 20 percent of all species on earth could be extinguished by the year 2000.[11]

At another level, the same destructive process can be seen in families whose members traditionally hide their differences for the sake of "keeping the peace." The more they keep their differences to themselves, the more secrets they keep, the more distance and distortion grows between them. Their days are marked by the suppression of intense feelings, and they make great efforts to dwell on the trivial so as to avoid the feared conflict. Yet, it has been my experience (and yours?) that when the secrets are out in the open, even though there is an explosion of intensity, people feel relieved and the family becomes stronger, more able to stand together in times of danger and joy. It appears that certain families have more of a tradition of intensity and willingness to face conflict openly. These characteristics are learned by the children and passed on to others. Unless the tradition of "keeping the (false) peace" is broken by family members who usually need help to do so, the marks of low intensity, avoidance of differences, and distance will continue in the history of the unfortunate family. After trying to help such a family, a helper is likely to come away with an overwhelming sense of loss and say, "What a waste!" Evil here is the loss of potential, a waste of possibilities. If more good is to be achieved in the lives of such families, unnecessary triviality must be overcome by creative intensity.

Griffin points to an important distinction between discord and triviality.[12] Discord results in physical or mental suffering, which is evil in itself without being compared to anything else or what might have been. There is some comfort in being told that things might have been worse when we suffer. We may even feel that we are better in some ways for having suffered. In my argument, however, this experience of good and evil is not the point. The word "intrinsic" points to a reality of good or evil apart from considerations of "for whom." From the standpoint of intrinsic good, it is always better if injury and suffering do not happen. The individual and the world would be better off without it. But the evil of triviality is different than the evil of discord in one respect. Triviality is evil by contrast to something else. Griffin says that an animal's existence is not evil because it is less intense than a human's. But when a human's life is reduced to that of an animal, one sees the evil of triviality. He continues, "Trivial experience is not evil just because it is trivial, it is evil only if it is more trivial than it had to be."[13]

When I recall what I was taught of the goodness of God, it was almost entirely on the side of prevention of harm (pain and suffering) done through discord. Could that be why you and I were so ready and poised to question the goodness of God? Griffin and Ogden point to a second kind of goodness that encourages ever more rewarding experiences, a good of a more positive kind. Something is added rather than only prevented. Increasing complexity overcomes unnecessary triviality. For more good—in the sense of increasingly richer experience—to be added to one's life, it is clear that bursts of intensity are needed to move from one stage of experience to another. Although a previous state of harmony may be disrupted by a new state of affairs, if sufficient intensity is available to "sort out" the new state of affairs, a new harmony follows that unites and completes the new situation.

What is biological evolution except one process among many that acts in and through them all, producing lavish variety and selecting for survival? Incredible patterns of harmony are laced with bursts of intensity by which new changes add to growth and development. Newer, more complex forms succeed older, simpler forms. This is the story of evolution. Wherever you look, the evolutionary pattern is visible. Evolution enhances the criteria of instrinsic goodness, harmony, and intensity. Evolution influences all other processes, including the religious process. You and I searched once for the meaning of life in the midst of a terrifying event. Would you agree that our relationship had a potential for growth, even from very humble beginnings?

Evolution is not God, although some thinkers see the ultimate meaning of life in evolution and feel there is no higher service than an ethics that serve the hidden purposes of evolution. Conrad Waddington devoted a large share of a great career in biology and science to this pursuit.[14] In my view, nothing, not even evolution, deserves the ultimate respect due to God alone. But you can hold, with no contradiction, that the limits of evolution are optimal because of God's creative work, without denying any evil that results from random changes in the genetic material, such as the one that affected your life and future. Further, you can hold that every good and evil, even in an evolving world, makes a difference to God, who continuously opens himself to the possibilities of richer and finer forms of goodness to be enjoyed by the creatures.

The Goodness of God and the Future of Genetic Disorders

Beyond the creative and redemptive characteristics of God's goodness, there is yet a third that directly helps you and everyone who ever felt punished by God because a genetic disorder was transmitted to a child. Schubert Ogden perceptively writes of the *emancipative* aspect of God's love, "whereby he intends the fullest possible self-realization of each of his creatures and infallibly acts to do all that can be done to that end save only what his creatures themselves have to do, both for themselves and for one another."[15] Creation and redemption are clearly the work of God alone, although we can participate in this work by witness, praise, worship, and thanksgiving. Only God holds together the cosmic order and provides the creative limits for all the forms and processes of life in the universe. Only God has the power to present this universe to each creature in every moment. Who else ought we to thank for a world in which more good than evil can be done? Further, only God is truly open to each being's struggle for freedom. Only God truly forgives our evasions of responsibility and harbors no desire to punish. Only God unfailingly recognizes the value of each creature in the total fabric of the universe. Who else ought we to thank for never forsaking any being in spite of the terrors of life and death? No one but God can do these mighty works.

God acts not only to save each creature from the terror of death in a physical sense, but also from the even deeper terror that life is meaningless due to the "perpetual perishing" of all. Everything relentlessly recedes into the past. Human memory is not sufficient to retain it all. Our fondest projects and ideals wither and die. Do you remember the words of the hymn, "Time like an ever-rolling stream bears all its sons away. They fly forgotten as a dream dies at the opening day"? I think of you often when singing these words. Your children are more quickly "borne away" by one of the many processes of time, evolution by natural selection. But, in truth, all of us sons and daughters of time are like small ships that were once moored by a rope to the bank of a mighty river. Our ships are launched when we are born. We are all being swept away, even as we make our lives, by the rivers of time that also help make us. Only God can save us and the world from perishing by accepting everything that is forevermore into his own life. Because everything that is affects God and he is open to all, nothing that is can be cast out into nothingness. The essence of faith is that the end of the journey, like the beginning, is firmly in the aim of God.

If God is mighty and good enough to save all from the most terrifying fate of making no difference whatsoever, it follows that God intends that all creatures be emancipated from any form of bondage that threatens to subvert the creative limits of natural order that allows a greater amount of good than evil to be realized. I believe that you can now see how a desire to be punished can be a form of bondage. We can enslave ourselves. Forms of bondage also include physical, social, or cultural arrangements that demean the freedom of all and prevent the fullest possible self-realization. Ogden recalls the cogent statement of St. Augustine that "he that made us without ourselves, will not save us without ourselves."[16] Unlike our response to God's work of creation and redemption, we must cooperate in the work of salvation more actively, because (as we have seen) not even God has the power totally to determine the being of others. Since everything has, in part, the power to determine itself, the life of creatures in the world is shaped by processes and decisions that are the result of creaturely freedom. There is no greater way to participate in God's work of salvation than to work for changes in ourselves, in society, and culture that enhance the process of emancipation from forms of bondage, as well as to be faithful companions to individuals who struggle for self-respect and freedom. Although God saves us by grace, we are also saved by faithful responses to opportunities to help ourselves and others realize our fullest human potential.

It is fair to say that a process of emancipation is underway as a result of new knowledge about genetics and opportunities to apply that knowledge to problems in society, including the possibility that human genetic disorders may be treatable in a primary, not only a secondary sense. A secondary treatment for Lesch-Nyhan disease, for example, may be found in a drug to reduce (even further) the damage done by so much uric acid, to act even better than the drug allopurinol does at present. Likewise, physicians prescribe diet therapies for disorders like galactosemia and PKU. But these are imperfect, in that they treat the product of the disorder and not the underlying cause. What if induced genetic changes were a better way to treat the faulty gene?

I am cautious but optimistic about research in human genetics. I do not confuse the search for new knowledge in genetics, or any type of research, with the work of God. God does not totally determine the pathways of research any more than the rivulets in the great stream of evolution. But it is not necessary to believe that human discovery makes no difference at all to God. There is no question but that research has enriched our lives. Why should we exclude God? Everything that is good affects God and is taken into God's life, making it richer. At quieter times, when I turn things over in my mind, I experiment with the notion that even God learns. When we work at the lab bench, or are at the patient's bedside, we can hold with no contradiction that we are engaged with God in a mighty work of emancipation. What we give to the research process is the courage to be truthful about the implications of knowledge, to be emancipated, as it were, from the bondage of old answers that no longer fit the questions. The unfailing strength to maintain the courage to be truthful, when it would be easier to accept a half-truth, is what God gives to the process of discovery. God does not forsake us in any time or place, but God does not do for us what we ought to do for ourselves.

We are being emancipated from inadequate answers to questions about how genes function and interact. There is a shroud of mystery around the whole area of genetics that is gradually being lifted.

Genes are being demystified. Genes are felt by some to belong only to God. A feeling of terror can accompany lifting the veil of mystery and peering into what was hitherto unknown. I say simply that there is no cause to be afraid of what we can discover about genes or about ourselves in the process of discovery. We should be more afraid of the consequences of avoiding discovery because we avoid conflicts between old and new answers.

We must not forget that, until only the last century, most people believed that genetic disorders, like all disease, were caused by supernatural forces. Not too many centuries ago, parents were persecuted and even killed because theories of demons and witches explained congenital malformations. Only in the last one hundred years, a very short time in the total scheme of things, have biological evolution and the laws of genetic inheritance come to be partially understood. Only in the past five years have the first genetic experiments been designed in animals that might be the forerunners of treatment in humans. You should especially keep your eye on experiments with mice that are bred with a form of thalassemia, a disease of hemoglobin, an element that helps make healthy red blood cells. Experiments are now underway to inject "borrowed cells" from humans, rabbits, and other mice directly into the fertilized eggs of mice that have the disease. The borrowed genes make hemoglobin correctly in the species from which they are taken. Scientists then implant the injected eggs into a mouse mother. They will see if the mouse offspring that might have died *in utero* due to the disease will be born alive as a result of the gene injection. The big question is whether the injection can be done early enough, before the message for incorrect hemoglobin "turns on" in the embryo.

Much more work needs to be done with animals for scientists to know enough about how borrowed genes function in a new location, whether any harm is done to other cells, and whether there are bad results, like cancer or other problems, in the offspring. Fortunately, mice have a very short gestation period and we can learn quickly from experiments. If a thalassemic mouse is cured, the next step would be to go to higher primates, including monkeys, who have the most physical similarities to humans. If this work succeeds, there will be a more solid scientific basis upon which to try the first medical experiment with humans to cure or prevent a genetic disorder.

What might that experiment look like? It could involve injecting segments of DNA that give the correct message to make hemoglobin, or in the case of Lesch-Nyhan disease, HGPRT. The most optimal time would probably be before the signal is given in the embryo for the particular gene to "turn on." Because it is possible to fertilize human eggs *in vitro* (since the birth of Louise Brown, the first so-called "test-tube" baby), perhaps the optimal time to experiment with treatment would be shortly after fertilization. Possibly there will be a test that one could do quickly to learn the sex and other information about the embryo. If the sex were male, in the instance of Lesch-Nyhan, there is a 50 percent risk of the disease. If no test existed to show if that particular embryo were destined to have the disease, treatment by injected genes could be tried and the embryo implanted in the mother. Perhaps there would be opportunities later to diagnose whether the disease still existed, and if further opportunities to treat presented themselves, it could be tried again.

If gene therapy does become scientifically feasible, in my view, it should be tried first in cases of very high risk genetic disorders, like Lesch-Nyhan and disease of the hemoglobin. The goal of human genetics should be primarily the search for better understanding of the ways and means to emancipate human beings from the burden of suffering brought on by random changes in genes. A mutant gene for Lesch-Nyhan disease or sickle cell disease is a form of bondage. These mutants are threats that more evil than good will exist for the affected persons. We need to be cautious about research in genetics, but we must not, in my view, neglect to do the great good that could be done if the scientific possibilities allow for it.

Not very long ago, a poor climate existed for research in human genetics. In the early 1970s, when scientists first recombined pieces of genes never before so combined (thus making a mutation), scientists were so cautious that they placed a voluntary moratorium on the work until stiff rules were in place that required extraordinary safety precautions to prevent biohazards. The media were full of stories about what has been called the "Frankenstein factor." Many people have a subliminal fear that new knowledge in genetics will lead to efforts to breed a super-race. I attended a meeting of geneti-

cists at the National Academy of Sciences in 1976 that was disrupted by protestors carrying signs accusing those who did DNA
recombinant research of Nazi thinking about eugenics and "Super-
man." One protestor's sign read, "Don't clone me." It was a difficult period for the study of human genetics. There was much
debate about how free scientists could be to pursue their goals.

In the years since 1975, when a voluntary moratorium was im-
posed, it has become clear that no hazards have emerged from this
research that were not already known; and, more important, no one
has been injured by any of the research. In a 1980 editorial in
Science, Maxine Singer, a molecular geneticist who had previously
regretted the voluntary moratorium because of the damage she felt
had been done to research, took a second look and changed her
mind. She wrote that "the cautious approach . . . continued by national guidelines in many countries, has not seriously hampered the
progress of research." She pointed to the manufacture of agents like
insulin and interferon by the use of DNA recombinant procedures
as the first fruits of genetic research. Then, in the most interesting
part of the editorial to me, she reviewed the basic insights into the
nature of genes that research had yielded.

> Once we thought the DNA of complex organisms was inscrutable . . .
> now we cope with it readily. . . .
> We thought of DNA as immovable, a fixed component of cells . . . now
> we know that some modules of DNA are peripatetic; their function de-
> pends on their ability to move around in a genome. . . .
> We thought genes were continuous stretches of DNA . . . now we know
> coding regions may be interrupted dozens of times, and spliced together in
> the form of messenger RNA when needed.
> We have learned that genes are fungible; animal genes function perfectly
> well within bacteria and bacterial genes within animal cells, confirming the
> unity of nature.
> We need no longer depend on chance events to generate the mutations
> essential for unraveling intricate genetic phenomena . . . specific mutations
> can be constructed at will, and millions of mutant genomes readily pro-
> duced for study.[17]

I find her thoughts very appealing, since they are a parallel in
science to the problem we faced in religion. She and her colleagues
thought that the DNA was inscrutable, immovable, perfectly con-

tinuous, uninterchangeable, and potentially dangerous to manipulate. You and I once thought that God was absolutely powerful, and absolutely incapable of being affected by good or evil. I hope that the cautious risk-taking that I have urged upon our ways of thinking about God's power and goodness lead to as much potential good for people who want their religious traditions to be related creatively to science as cautious risk-taking in human genetics appears to hold for the alleviation of genetic disorders. Could there be something more than simple parallelism in these two possibilities?

Let me say it plainly. I believe that the pain and suffering that you experienced was not lost in the rivers of time. Your suffering makes a difference to God, who not only gives unfailing courage to face the unknown, but who also creates the limits of our freedom to learn in such a way that more good than evil can eventually prevail. If a child is ever cured of a genetic disorder by a gene therapy that is the result of scientific research, the event will not have removed the evil that was done to you and your family. But you and I will have understood more about the goodness of God and the meaning of participation in God's emancipating work. God's abiding intent is emancipation and not punishment.

Appendix A. Glossary of Terms and Common Genetic Disorders

Allele. Alleles are different forms of a gene in the same place on paired chromosomes. They segregate at meiosis. A child normally receives only one of each pair of alleles from each parent.

Amino acids. The building blocks of protein, for which DNA forms the genetic code.

Amniocentesis. Needle puncture of the uterus and amniotic cavity through the abdominal wall to allow amniotic fluid to be withdrawn by syringe. The term is often applied to the whole procedure of prenatal diagnosis by culture and analysis of amniotic fluid cells.

Beta-thalassemia. See *Thalassemia*.

Birth defect. A disease, disorder, or other condition present at birth that can impair an individual's health.

Carrier. An individual who carries one normal gene and one abnormal gene. The person may look and feel normal. If that person mates with another carrier, there is a one in four risk of conceiving an affected child.

Cell. The living active microscopic unit of all plants and animals, consisting of many specialized parts.

Chromosome abnormality, or error. An abnormality of chromosome number or structure.

This material is adapted from pp. 72–78 of *Genetic Conditions* (1977), published by the California State Department of Education, and used with permission.

Chromosomes. Microscopic threadlike bodies in the nuclei of cells.

Cleft lip/palate. Symptoms: immediately observable at birth. Cleft lip: failure of two sides of the upper lip to grow together properly. Cleft palate: a split or opening in the roof of the mouth leading to complications in breathing, speech, hearing, and ingestion of food. These conditions occur both together and separately. Treatment: corrective surgery, speech therapy. Pattern of transmission: variable, often multifactorial.

Clone. A cell line derived by mitosis from a single ancestral cell.

Club foot. Symptoms: twisted position of one or both of a baby's feet, easily recognizable at birth, resulting, if untreated, in inability to walk and/or shortened legs or toes. Treatment: surgery, corrective shoes or braces. With proper care, most affected individuals can walk normally by the time they reach physical maturity. Pattern of transmission: multifactorial.

Congenital defect. A defect present at birth; it may be determined genetically or by external influences during intrauterine life.

Consanguinity. A characteristic of two or more individuals if they have a common recent ancestor (usually not more remote than three or four generations).

Congenital trait. Trait present at birth, not necessarily genetic.

Cystic fibrosis. Symptoms: unusually thick mucus blocks the lungs, causing coughing, difficult breathing, infections, and distended lungs. Secretion of the digestive juices is reduced, causing poor digestion of food, a massive appetite, thin body build, poor tolerance of exercise, short stature, and in some cases delayed sexual maturation. Salt is lost in perspiration more easily than normally. Treatment: life expectancy is shorter than normal. Physical therapy can improve breathing; synthetic digestive enzymes can improve digestion; salt tablets can help to avoid loss of salt in perspiration; antibiotics can treat lung infections. Pattern of transmission: Recessive.

Cytology. The study of cells.

Cytogenetics. The study of the genetic effects of cellular reproduction, focusing primarily on the chromosomes.

Deletion. Loss of part of a chromosome.

Diabetes. Symptoms: thirst, increased appetite, weakness, weight loss; in extreme circumstances, unconsciousness or convulsions. Treatment: since diabetes is essentially the result of metabolic disorders leading to high blood sugar, this condition can be corrected by insulin injections and careful diet and exercise. Pattern of transmission: multifactorial.

Diploid. The number of chromosomes in most body cells, which is double the number in the sex cells. In human beings, the diploid chromosome number is forty-six.

Dizygotic (dizygous). Refers to twins derived from separate eggs ("fraternal twins").

DNA. Deoxyribonucleic acid, the nucleic acid of the chromosomes.

Dominance. The quality of a particular trait that appears when it is paired genetically with a different trait, the second trait being recessive.

Down syndrome. Symptoms: in early stages of development, distinct physical features: slanting eyes (Down syndrome is sometimes referred to as "mongolism"), curving folds of skin at the eyes, shorter than average stature, often a single large crease on the palm of the hand. In later stages of development, varying degrees of mental retardation, occasionally heart disease and other complications. Treatment: antibiotics for some complications attending Down syndrome; special education. Life expectancy may be nearly normal. Pattern of transmission: chromosome abnormality.

Dysgenic. Due to, or determining, an increase in the frequency of deleterious genes. Dysgenic effects may be spontaneous, or they may result from medical or social interventions that improve the fitness of the handicapped.

Environment. The conditions or influences present in the world an individual inhabits.

Eugenics. Improving human beings by the deliberate selection of certain types of people to perpetuate their qualities.

Euthenics. Improving human beings through changes in the environment.

Evolution. Gradual change from one form to a new, or different, form.

Fetoscopy. A technique for direct visualization of the fetus used for prenatal diagnosis.

Fetus. The developing organism of a human being prior to birth.

Fitness, Darwinian. Measured by reproductive performance, that is, number of offspring. The average is considered a fitness of 1.

Gamete. A reproductive cell (ovum or sperm) with a haploid chromosome number.

Genes. The units in chromosomes that determine hereditary traits.

Genetic condition. Any quality or trait that an individual inherits from his or her parents.

Genetic code. The process of chemical change and recombination that occurs during cell division, involving the four basic chemical compounds of DNA and the twenty amino acids that make up all proteins.

Genetic death. Failure of the individual to reproduce.

Genetic screening. A systematic testing of persons designed to detect potential genetic handicaps in them or in their progeny, particularly those who may respond to treatment.

Genetic trait. Trait determined by genes, not necessarily congenital.

Genetics. The scientific study of heredity.

Genome. The total genetic endowment.

Genotype. The genetic constitution, either at one specific location of a gene or more generally. In the general sense, genotype is essentially synonymous with genome. *See* Phenotype.

Haploid. The chromosome number of a normal gamete (sperm or ovum) containing only one chromosome of each type. In human beings, the haploid number is twenty-three.

Hemophilia. Symptoms: poor clotting of blood, spontaneous bleeding or excessive bleeding after minor injury; damage to joints. Treatment: injections of the deficient clotting factor. With proper care, hemophiliacs can lead normal lives, although they must take care in exercising. Pattern of transmission: X-linked.

Heredity. The inheritance of physical and mental characteristics.

Heterozygote. An individual who has two different alleles, one of which is the normal allele, the other, abnormal, at a given position on a pair of homologous chromosomes.

Homologous chromosomes. A "matched pair" of chromosomes, one from each parent, having the same gene position in the same order.

Homozygote. An individual possessing a pair of identical abnormal alleles at a given position on a pair of homologous chromosomes.

Huntington's disease. Symptoms: between the ages of thirty and forty, progressive deterioration of the brain and central nervous system, producing involuntary jerking, loss of mental abilities, depression, insanity, and ultimately death. Treatment: none. Pattern of transmission: dominant.

Hydrocephalus. Symptoms: larger than normal size head. Hydrocephalus is the result of abnormal quantities of cerebrospinal fluid in the brain, usually due to a blockage, tumor, or malformation that interferes with the circulation of the fluid through the central nervous system. Treatment: surgical removal of excess fluid. Without treatment, affected children rarely survive. Pattern of transmission: multifactorial.

Inborn error. A genetically determined biochemical disorder in which a specific enzyme defect produces a metabolic block that may have pathological consequences.

Klinefelter syndrome. When a child is born with Y chromosome and two or more X chromosomes. Results in a sexually underdeveloped male with minor malformations and varying degrees of mental deficiency.

Lesch-Nyhan syndrome. A hereditary disorder that occurs only in males. Symptoms: high concentrations of uric acid in the blood, abnormal movements of the body, mental retardation, and involuntary biting of the lips and fingers. The disorder is associated with a failure to form an enzyme necessary for purine synthesis. Treatment: none (most affected boys die by their teens). Pattern of transmission: X-linked.

Meiosis. The special type of cell division occurring in the germ cells.

Mitosis. The reproduction of a cell by dividing into an exact duplicate of itself.

Multifactorial. Determined by multiple factors, genetic and nongenetic, yet in a discernible hereditary fashion.

Muscular dystrophy. Symptoms: muscular dystrophy is actually a group of disorders, all of which involve damage to the muscles supporting the skeleton, resulting in progressive weakness. Duchenne-type muscular dystrophy, occurring in the first few years of life, is the most common. Treatment: temporary relief through therapy and braces. Death usually occurs within fifteen to twenty years of onset. Pattern of transmission: commonly X-linked.

Mutagen. A physical or chemical agent that increases the mutation rate.

Mutation. A failure of a gene to produce an exact self-copy, resulting in modification of the hereditary trait produced by that gene.

Nucleus. The central part of a cell.

Phenotype. The observable characteristics of the organism. The distinction between genotype (which see) and phenotype is similar to that between character and reputation.

Phenylketonuria (PKU). Symptoms: an inborn error of metabolism, PKU is the inability to metabolize the amino acid phenylalanine. In the newborn, PKU can be detected through a simple blood test. Later on, a child with PKU can be identified by unusually lighter hair or skin than his or her siblings. In advanced stages, PKU can produce abnormal destructive behavior and degrees of mental retardation. Treatment: The most serious effects of PKU can be prevented in infancy through a special diet that balances the body's lack of the phenylalanine enzyme. If PKU advances beyond this stage, institutionalization may be required to deal with severe mental and physical retardation. Pattern of transmission: recessive.

Prenatal care. Maintenance of a mother's health prior to the birth of her child.

Prenatal diagnosis. Determination of the likelihood of birth defects in an unborn fetus.

Proband. The affected individual who first comes to attention and brings the family to study.

Psychomotor. Of or relating to motor action directly proceeding from mental activity.

Recessiveness. The quality of a particular trait that does not appear when paired genetically with a dominant trait.

Recombination. The formation of new combinations of linked genes by crossing-over between their positions.

Rh incompatibility. Symptoms: in the newborn child, jaundice, anemia, stillbirth, or complications leading to mental retardation and subnormal physical development. Treatment: Rh disease is the result of the incompatibility of Rh blood factors in the mother and father. Although once among the most common cause of birth defects, the disease can now be prevented completely by a vaccine developed in 1968. Pattern of transmission: Dominant. Rh factor disease can occur only in situations where the father has Rh positive blood while the mother has Rh negative blood.

Sex chromosomes. Chromosomes responsible for sex determination.

Sex-linked. Usually refers to a disorder determined by a gene located on the X chromosome. Although a Y-linked trait is also sex-linked, X-linked is the preferable term.

Sickle cell disease. Symptoms: a blood test will reveal that the bearer of this disease has blood cells that are sickle-shaped, rather than the normal round shape. Although victims of this disease can lead normal lives, severe anemia is common, and affected individuals experience periodic pain and infections. The life span is shorter than normal. Treatment: no cure has been found. Temporary analgesic relief, antibiotics, and occasional blood transfusions are necessary. Pattern of transmission: recessive.

Species. Groups of living organisms that interbreed.

Sperm. Male germ (sex) cells that unite with female ova (egg) cells to produce a new organism.

Spina bifida. Symptoms: a defect in the bone structure of the spinal column, often producing a large cyst containing parts of the spinal cord, observable at birth. Treatment: corrective surgery. In severe cases, children who have been treated are paralyzed below the waist. Pattern of transmission: multifactorial.

Tay-Sachs disease. Symptoms: an infant with Tay-Sachs disease appears normal at birth. Within four to eight months, the first symptoms appear in the form of weakness, sluggishness, and poor psychomotor development. The symptoms become progressively more severe—blindness, deafness, seizures, paralysis, and total mental retardation usually occur. Death always occurs by three to five years of age. Treatment: none. Pattern of transmission: recessive.

Thalassemia (Cooley's anemia). Symptoms: Severe anemia, the result of a failure of the body to produce blood cells with the normal amount of hemoglobin. Children with thalassemia are pale and listless. Treatment: hemoglobin transfusions throughout life, beginning in the first year. Pattern of transmission: Recessive.

Trait. Any gene-determined characteristic. Although in medicine it has come to be used particularly for the heterozygous state of a recessive disorder such as sickle cell disease, it has a more general meaning in genetics.

Trisomy. Three chromosomes of one type in a person. The commonest in humans is trisomy 21 (Down syndrome).

Turner syndrome. Child born with only one X chromosome, and is missing either another X chromosome or a Y chromosome needed to fully define sex. Results in a sexually underdeveloped female, with stunted growth and sometimes mild mental deficiency.

Zygote. The primordial cell of a new organism, formed by the fusion of an egg and a sperm.

Appendix B. Conditions That Can Be (I) Diagnosed Prenatally, (II) Diagnosed in the Newborn, (III) Screened in the Carrier State

I

Abruptio placentae
Acardia
Acephalus
Achondrogenesis
Achondroplasia
Acid phosphatase deficiency
Acute intermittent porphyria
Adenosine deaminase deficiency
Adrenogenital syndrome
Agnathia-microstomia-synotia
  syndrome
Albert-Schönberg disease
Amelia

Aminopterin syndrome
Amniocele
Amniotic adhesion malformation
  complex
Amniotic band disruption complex
Amniotic band syndrome
Anal atresia
Anencephaly
Antral diaphragm
Argininosuccinic aciduria
Arrhythmia, cardiac
Arthrogryposis
Ascites
Asphyxiating thoracic dystrophy
Atresia of lymphatic system

This material is adapted from Sharon Stephenson and David Weaver, "Prenatal Diagnosis: A Compilation of Diagnosed Conditions," *American Journal of Obstetrics and Gynecology* 141 (1981), pp. 319–343.

Beckwith-Wiedemann syndrome
Bermann disease
Bilateral renal agenesis
Bladder distension
Blighted ovum
Body wall defects with reduction
   limb anomalies
Bradycardia
Calcified umbilical cord
Campomelic dysplasia
Campomelic dwarfism
Caudal regression syndrome
Chondroectodermal dysplasia
Chorioangioma
Chromosomal anomalies, general
Chronic granulomatous disease
Chylothorax
Classic hemophilia
Cleft lip
Cleft palate
Cleidocranial dysplasia
Clover-leaf skull
Combined immunodeficiency
   disease
Complete heart block
Congenital adrenal hyperplasia
Congenital bullous ichthyosiform
   erythroderma
Congenital coxa vara
Congenital hydrocele
Congenital ichthyosis
Congenital nephrosis
Congenital nephrotic syndrome
Conjoined twins
Cranioachischisis
Craniosynostosis
Cretinism
Cystic dysplastic kidney
Cystic fibrosis
Cystic hygroma

Cystic lymphangioma
Cystinosis
Cystinuria
Cytomegalovirus infection
Dandy-Walker syndrome
Diabetic embryopathy syndrome
Diaphragmatic hernia
Down syndrome
Duchenne muscular dystrophy
Duodenal atresia
Dysplastic kidney
Dystrophia myotonica
Eagle-Barrett syndrome
Ectopic fetal liver
Ectopic pregnancy
Ectromelia
Ellis-van Creveld syndrome
EMG syndrome
Encephalocele
Enteric cyst
Epidermolysis bullosa letalis
Epidermolysis bullosa simplex
Epidermolytic hyperkeratosis
Epignathus
Erythroblastosis fetalis
Esophageal atresia
Exomphalos
Exomphalos-macroglossia-gigantism
   syndrome
Fabry disease
Familial hypercholesterolemia
Fanconi anemia
Farber disease
Fetal ascites
Fetal demise
Fetal fracture secondary to
   maternal abdominal trauma
Fetal growth deficiency
Fetal hydrops
Fetal ovarian cyst

Fetal rickets
Fetus papyraceous
Galactose-1-phosphate uridyl
  transferase deficiency
Galactosemia
Gangliosidosis, Gm$_1$-type 1
Gangliosidosis, Gm$_1$-type 2
Gastric obstruction
Gastroschisis
Gaucher disease
Globoid cell leukodystrophy
Glucose phosphate isomerase
  deficiency
Glutaric acidemia
Glycogenosis type II
Golding deformity
Harlequin ichthyosis
Heart block
Hemangioma
Hemoglobin H disease
Hemophilia A
Herpes type I infection
Holoprosencephaly
Homocystinuria
Homozygous achondroplasia
Hunter syndrome
Hurler syndrome
Hydramnios
Hydranencephaly
Hydrocele
Hydrocephalus
Hydronephrosis
Hydrops fetalis
21-Hydroxylase deficiency
Hygroma
Hypercholesterolemia
Hyperthyroidism
Hypophosphatasia
Hypoplastic right ventricle
Hypothyroidism

Hypoxanthine-guanine
  phosphoribosyl transferase
  deficiency
I-cell disease
Ichthyosis congenita
Iniencephaly
Intrathoracic cyst
Intrauterine fetal death
Intrauterine growth retardation
Ivemark syndrome
Jarcho-Levin syndrome
Jejunal atresia
Jeune syndrome
Ketotic hyperglycinemia
Krabbe disease
Lemellar ichthyosis
Lesch-Nyhan syndrome
Lipogranulomatosis, familial
Lung tumor
Lymphangiectasia
Lymphedema
Lysosomal acid phosphatase
  deficiency
Macroglossia-omphalocele-viscero-
  megaly syndrome
Maroteaux-Lamy syndrome
Meckel syndrome
Meckel-Gruber syndrome
Meconium ileus
Meconium peritonitis
Megacystis-microcolon-intestinal
  hypoperistalsis syndrome
Megaureter
Meningocele
Meningomyelocele
Menke disease
Metachromatic leukodystrophy
Methylmalonic
  aciduria-5'-Deoxyadenosyl-cobala-
  min deficiency

Methylmalonic CoA mutase deficiency
Microcephaly
Molar pregnancy
Mucolipidosis type II
Mucolipidosis type IV
Mucopolysaccharidosis type I H
Mucopolysaccharidosis type II
Mucopolysaccharidosis type III A
Mucopolysaccharidosis type VI
Mucoviscidosis
Multicystic kidney disease
Muscular dystrophy
Myelocele
Myelomeningocele
Myotonic dystrophy
Necrosis of fetal liver
Nephrosis
Neuraminidase deficiency
Niemann-Pick Disease, type A
Nonbullous congenital ichthyosiform erythrodermia
Nuchal bleb
Nuchal lymphangiectasia
Occipito-facial-cervico-thoracic-abdomino-digital dysplasia
Oligodactyly
Oligohydramnios
Omphalocele
Osteogenesis imperfecta congenita
Osteogenesis imperfecta tarda
Osteopetrosis
Osteopoikilie
Otocephaly
Ovarian cyst
Pericardial effusion
Phocomelia
Pilonidal sinus
Pituitary hormone deficiency
Placenta previa

Placental steroid sulfatase deficiency
Placental tumor
Placentomegaly
Polycystic kidneys
Polyhydramnios
Pompe disease
Posterior fossa cyst
Potter syndrome
Primary pituitary dysgenesis
Propionic acidemia
Proximal femoral dysplasia
Prune-belly syndrome
Rachischisis
Radius, absent
Renal agenesis
Renal cysts
Rickets
Roberts syndrome
Rubella infection
Sacral agenesis
Saldino-Noonan dwarfism
Sandhoff disease
Sanfilippo syndrome A
Short rib-polydactyly syndrome, Saldino-Noonan type
Short rib-polydactyly syndrome, Spranger-Verma type
Sialidosis
Siamese twins
Sickle cell anemia
Sirenomelia
Skull fracture
Small for gestational age
Spina bifida cystica
Spina bifida occulta
Spondylothoracic dysplasia
Spotted bones
Steinert syndrome
Steroid sulfatase deficiency

Streeter bands
Symmelia
Syphilis infection
Tachycardia
TAR syndrome
Tay-Sachs disease
Teratoma—brain
Teratoma—mouth
Teratoma—neck
Teratoma—sacrococcygeal
Tetralogy of Fallot
alpha-Thalassemia
beta-Thalassemia
Thantophoric dwarfism
Thoracic cyst
Thrombocytopenia-absent radii
  syndrome
Thyroid tumor
Thyrotoxicosis
Triad syndrome
Tricuspid atresia
Triploidy
Trisomy 13
Trisomy 18
Trisomy 21
Tumor—lung
Tumor—placenta
Tumor—thyroid
Turner syndrome
Ureteral obstruction with cystic
  dysplastic kidney
Urethral obstruction malformation
  complex
Ventricle, hypoplastic right
Ventricular enlargement, heart
Vitamin D deficient rickets
Werdnig-Hoffman disease,
  group 1
Wiedemann-Beckwith syndrome
Wolman disease

X-linked hydrocephalus
Xeroderma pigmentosum

II

Amino Acid Disorders
Argininosuccinic aciduria
Cystathioninuria
Cystinuria
Fanconi syndrome
Histidinemia
Hyperglycinemia
Hyperlysinemia
Hyperornithinemia
Hyperphenylalaninemia without
  PKU
Homocystinuria

Carbohydrate Disorders
Galactosemia

Red Blood Cell Disorders
Glucose-6-phosphate
  dehydrogenase deficiency
  (G-6-PD)
Sickle cell disorder

Immunologic or Related
Disorders
Angioneurotic edema, hereditary
  (HANE)
Alpha one-antitrypsin deficiency

Iminoglycinuria   **III***
Maple sugar urine
   disease   Beta- and alpha-thalassemia trait
Phenylketonuria (PKU)   Sickle cell trait
Tyrosinemia (tyrosinosis)   Tay-Sachs carrier trait

---

*The recessive traits listed here can be detected in the carrier state by simple blood tests with a high degree of accuracy. Tests are being designed to identify carriers of other common genetic disorders. Counselors and parents should keep abreast of reports on tests for recessive genes in carriers of the trait for chronic granulomatosis, cystic fibrosis, Duchenne muscular dystrophy, hemophilia, Lesch-Nyhan disease, metachromatic leukodystrophy, ornithine transcaramylase deficiency, phenylketonuria, and X-linked recessive mental retardation.

Appendix C. Family Health History Chart with Instructions for Use

A family health history is an important part of your health record. It can be helpful in the early diagnosis and treatment of disease and is indispensable for genetic counseling. In attempting to outline your family history, take a moment to think about your family as a whole. If possible, talk to others in the family to confirm or add to what you know.

In addition to the more common disorders, such as diabetes, high blood pressure, heart disease, and cancer, are there any conditions that are found in several or more members of your family? Note any individuals with severe or long-lasting illnesses or disabilities. Is there anyone who is mentally retarded or mentally ill? Investigate the early death of a child or adult. Record any history of miscarriages or repeated abortions. Note the geographical region from which your family stemmed several generations back. Were there any cousin marriages and, if so, when?

Start your history with the immediate family, but include as much of the extended family—aunts, uncles, cousins—as you can. Here is an outline to guide you in recording such information.

Modeled after the March of Dimes Birth Defects Foundation Family Medical Record.

Name	Date of Birth	Health History (Include major illness[es], hospitalization[s], use of medications, allergies, special problems)	Age and Cause of Death
HUSBAND (Blood type)			
His father			
His mother			
His brothers and sisters and their children			
His grandfather			
His grandmother			
His aunts and uncles and their children			

Additional information

Family Physician(s)

Location of Pertinent Medical Records

Name	Date of Birth	Health History (Include major illness[es], hospitalization[s], use of medications, allergies, special problems)	Age and Cause of Death
WIFE (Blood type)			
Her father			
Her mother			
Her brothers and sisters and their children			
Her grandfather			
Her grandmother			
Her aunts and uncles and their children			

Additional information

_____

Family Physician(s)

_____

Location of Pertinent Medical Records

_____

Name	Date of Birth	Description (Include brief history of labor and delivery [including hospital and M.D.'s], birth weight and condition at birth, growth and development, current status)
CHILD(REN)		

Notes

Chapter 1

1. Aubrey Milunsky, *Know Your Genes* (Boston: Houghton Mifflin, 1977), p. 1.
2. Richard Dawkins, *The Selfish Gene* (New York: Oxford University Press, 1976), p. 23.
3. Dawkins, *The Selfish Gene*, p. 24.
4. James D. Watson, *The Double Helix* (New York: Atheneum Publishers, 1968).
5. Milunsky, *Know Your Genes*, p. 109.
6. Ron Davidson, "Problems in Genetic Screening," *Social Issues in Human Genetics* (Ottawa: Science Council of Canada, 1980). 100 Metcalfe St., Ottawa, Ontario, KI P 5M1.
7. R.L. Nalbaldian, "Mass Screening Programs for Sickle Cell Hemoglobin," *Journal of the American Medical Association* 221 (1972), p. 500.
8. Research Group of Ethical, Social, and Legal Issues in Genetic Counseling and Genetic Engineering, "Ethical and Social Issues in Screening for Genetic Disease," *New England Journal of Medicine* 286 (1972), p. 1129.
9. Milunsky, *Know Your Genes*, p. 94.
10. Leonard A. Herzenberg, et al., "Fetal Cells in the Blood of Pregnant Women: Detection and Enriching by Fluorescence-Activating Cell Sorting," *Proceedings of the National Academy of Science* 76 (1979), p. 1453.
11. Sherman Elias and Maurice J. Mahoney, "Prenatal Diagnosis of Trisomy 13 with Decision Not to Terminate Pregnancy," *Obstetrics and Gynecology* 47 (1976), pp. 75–76.
12. Michael R. Harrison, et al, "Management of the Fetus with a Urinary Tract Malformation," *Journal of the American Medical Association* 246 (1981), pp. 635–639.
13. Michael R. Harrison, et al., "Fetal Surgery for Congenital Hydronephrosis," *New England Journal of Medicine* 306 (1982), pp. 591–593.
14. Michael R. Harrison, Mitchell S. Golbus, and Roy A. Filly, "Management of the Fetus with a Correctable Congenital Defect," *Journal of the American Medical Association* 246 (1981), pp. 772–773; and John C. Fletcher, "The Fetus as Patient: Ethical Issues," *Journal of the American Medical Association* 246 (1981), pp. 772–773.

15. This case was prepared from "Report of the National Institutes of Health Ad Hoc Committee on the UCLA Report Concerning Certain Research Activities of Dr. Martin J. Cline," May 21, 1981. Another public report of the case can be found in Gina Bari Kolata and Nicholas Wade, "Human Gene Treatment Stirs New Debate," *Science* 210 (1980), p. 407.

Chapter 2

1. Constant H. Jacquet, Jr. (ed.), *Yearbook of American and Canadian Churches* (Nashville: Abingdon Press, 1981), pp. 232–236.
2. David S. Schuller, Merton P. Strommen, and Milo L. Brekke (eds.), *Ministry in America* (San Francisco: Harper & Row, 1980), pp. 79–89.
3. Erik H. Erikson, *Young Man Luther* (New York: W. W. Norton and Company, 1962), p. 118.
4. Peter Berger and Thomas Luckman, *The Social Construction of Reality* (Garden City, New York: Doubleday, 1966); and Peter Berger, *The Sacred Canopy-Elements of a Sociological Theory of Religion* (Garden City, New York: Doubleday, 1967).
5. Ernest Becker, *The Denial of Death* (New York: The Free Press, 1973), p. 54.
6. Gerhard Kittel (ed.), *Theological Dictionary of the New Testament*, vol. 1, trans. Geoffrey W. Bromley (Grand Rapids, Michigan: Wm. B. Eerdmans, 1964), pp. 232–233, 271, 335 f.
7. *The Interpreter's Bible*, vol. 7 (New York: Abingdon-Cokesbury Press, 1951), p. 772.
8. For my thoughts on this subject, see John C. Fletcher, "Trends in the Futures of Theological Seminaries" (Washington, D.C.: The Alban Institute, 1982).
9. John C. Fletcher, "Religious Authenticity in the Clergy" (Washington, D.C.: The Alban Institute, 1975).
10. Bruce Reed, *Dynamics of Religion: Process and Movement in Christian Churches* (London: Darton, Longman, and Todd, Ltd., 1978); John C. Harris, *Stress, Power, and Ministry* (Washington, D.C.: Alban Institute, 1977); and James R. Adams and Celia A. Hahn, *Learning to Share the Ministry* (Washington, D.C.: The Alban Institute, 1975).

Chapter 3

1. National Center for Health Statistics, Public Health Service, *First Marriages, United States, 1968–1976*, DHEW Publication No. (PHS) 79-1913, p. 5.
2. Lawrence Stone, "The Rise of the Nuclear Family in Early Modern England: The Patriarchal Stage," in Charles E. Rosenberg (ed.), *The Family in History* (Philadelphia: University of Pennsylvania Press, 1975), pp. 12–57.
3. There is ample evidence of the great social and psychological stress on the marriages of couples who have children with serious malformations. I collected some of this literature in "Attitudes Toward Defective Newborns," *Hastings Center Studies* 2 (1974), pp. 21–32. There is no reliable study on the divorce rate among such couples in the United States, but it is perceived to be higher than among other couples by practitioners. A 1971 British study that followed four hundred couples who sought genetic counseling after the birth of an affected child found a divorce rate twice the average. Cedric O. Carter, K. A. Evans, J. A. Fraser Roberts, and A. R. Buck, "Genetic Clinic: A Follow-Up Study," *Lancet*, Feb. 6, 1971, pp. 281–285. It is likely that the divorce rate varies with the disease. For parents in twenty-nine families children with cystic fibrosis, the divorce rate

is the same as the national average; cf. Michael L. Begleiter, V. F. Burry, and David J. Harris, "Prevalence of Divorce Among Parents of Children with Cystic Fibrosis and Other Chronic Diseases," *Social Biology* 23 (1976), pp. 260–264. In Great Britain, the divorce rate for 142 families with a child born with a neural tube defect was nine times higher than that of the local population; cf. B. J. Tew, K. M. Lawrence, H. Payne, and K. Rawnsley, "Marital Stability Following the Birth of a Child with Spina Bifida," *British Journal of Psychiatry* 131 (1977), pp. 79–82.

4. Murray Bowen, *Family Therapy in Clinical Practice* (New York: Aronson, 1978); and John G. Howells, *Theory and Practice of Family Psychiatry* (New York: Brunner/Mazel Publishers, 1971), p. 34.

5. Aubrey Milunsky, *Know Your Genes,* (Boston: Houghton Mifflin, 1977) p. 53.

6. This case was provided by Sandra L. Schlesinger, M.S., Genetic Counselor, Institute Genetics Program, Clinical Center, NIH, Bethesda, Md.

7. David M. Feldman, "Eugenics and Religious Law: Jewish Religious Laws," *Encyclopedia of Bioethics*, vol. 1, edited by Warren T. Reich (New York: Free Press, 1978), p. 469.

8. Josef Warkany, "Congenital Malformations of the Past," *Journal of Chronic Diseases* 10 (1959), p. 84f.; and Josef Warkany, *Congenital Malformations* (Chicago: Year Book Medical Publishers, 1971).

9. Tom L. Beauchamp and James F. Childress, *Principles of Biomedical Ethics* (New York: Oxford University Press, 1979), pp. 97–134.

10. I am grateful to Ruth Faden, Larry McCullough, and Joseph McInerney for the use of this case.

11. James J. Lynch, *The Broken Heart: The Medical Consequences of Loneliness* (New York: Basic Books, 1977).

Chapter 4

1. Albert R. Jonsen and George Lister, "Newborn Intensive Care: The Ethical Problems," *Hastings Center Report* 8 (1978), p. 15.

2. A. L. Villumsen, "Environmental Factors in Congenital Abnormality," *Obstetrical and Gynecological Survey* 26 (1971), pp. 635–637.

3. M. J. Konner, "Aspects of the Development Ethology of a Foraging People," in N. B. Jones (ed.), *Ethological Studies of Child Behavior* (London: Cambridge University Press, 1972).

4. Aron Bentovim, "Emotional Disturbances of Handicapped Pre-School Children and Their Families: Attitudes Toward the Child," *British Medical Journal* 2 (1972), pp. 579–581.

5. Marshall H. Klaus and John H. Kennell, *Maternal-Infant Bonding* (St. Louis: C. V. Mosby Company, 1976), p. 169.

6. G. H. Zuk, "Religious Factor and Role of Guilt in Parental Acceptance of the Retarded Child," *American Journal of Mental Deficiency* 64 (1959), pp. 139–147.

7. Alfred L. Lazar, Russell E. Orpet, and Virgil A. Revie, "Attitudes of Young Gifted Boys and Girls Toward Handicapped Individuals," *Exceptional Children* 38 (1972), pp. 489–490.

8. Nancy A. Irvin, John H. Kennell, and Marshall H. Klaus, "Caring for Parents of an Infant with a Congenital Malformation," in Klaus and Kennell, *Maternal-Infant Bonding*, p. 182.

9. Bruno Bettelheim, "How Do You Help a Child Who Has a Physical Handicap?" *Ladies Home Journal* 89 (1972), pp. 34–35.

10. Hannah Arendt, *The Human Condition* (Chicago: University of Chicago Press, 1959), p. 222.
11. Robert J. Lifton and E. Olson, *Living and Dying* (New York: Praeger, 1974), p. 82.
12. John C. Fletcher, "Parents in Genetic Counseling: The Moral Shape of Decisionmaking," in *Ethical Issues in Human Genetics,* edited by Bruce Hilton, Daniel Callahan, et al. (New York: Plenum Press, 1973), p. 319.
13. For such a discussion, see my chapter "Is Euthanasia Ever Justifiable?" in *Controversies in Oncology,* edited by Peter Wiernick (New York: Wiley, 1982), pp. 297–321.
14. Bok's ethical position against infanticide requires no special religious appeal to back it up; cf. Sisela Bok, "Ethical Problems of Abortion," *Hasting Center Studies* 2 (1974) pp. 42–44.
15. John H. Kennell, et al., "The Mourning Response of Parents to the Death of a Newborn Infant," *New England Journal of Medicine* 283 (1970) pp. 344–349.
16. Raymond S. Duff, "On Deciding the Use of the Family Commons," in *Birth Defects: Original Article Series,* 12 (1976), pp. 73–84.
17. Klaus and Kennell, *Maternal-Infant Bonding,* p. 212.
18. Kennell et al., "The Mourning Responses," p. 345.
19. Renee C. Fox and Judith P. Swazey, *The Courage to Fail* (Chicago: University of Chicago Press, 1974), p. 322.
20. This interview with David Abramson, M.D., conducted in 1974, was first published in my article "Spina Bifida with Myelomeningocele: A Case Study in Attitudes Towards Defective Newborns" in C. Swinyard, ed., *Decision-making and Defective Newborn* (Springfield: Charles C. Thomas, 1978), p. 300. Courtesy of David C. Abramson and Charles C. Thomas, Publisher, Springfield, Illinois.

Chapter 5

1. Erik Erikson, "The Healthy Personality," *Psychological Issues* (monograph), vol. 1 (1959), p. 59.
2. T. S. Eliot, "Burnt Norton," *Four Quartets* (New York: Harcourt Brace Jovanovich and London: Faber and Faber, Ltd., 1968), p. 3.
3. Although I am responsible for the content of this section on the ethical process and accountability, I have drawn on the work of two moral philosophers who wrote about it long before I put these thoughts together. Henry David Aiken, *Reason and Conduct* (New York: Knopf, 1962), pp. 75–82; and H. Richard Niebuhr, *The Responsible Self* (New York: Harper & Row, 1963), pp. 64–65.
4. Niebuhr, *The Responsible Self,* p. 108.

Chapter 6

1. Bruce D. Blumberg, Mitchell S. Golbus, and Karl H. Hanson, "The Psychological Sequelae of Abortion Performed for a Genetic Indication," *American Journal of Obstetrics and Gynecology* 122 (1975), pp. 799–808.
2. John C. Fletcher, "The Brink: The Parent-Child Bond in the Genetic Revolution," *Theological Studies* 33 (1972), pp. 496–477.

Chapter 7

1. Paul Ricoeur, *The Symbolism of Evil* (Boston: Beacon Press, 1967), p. 31.
2. Alfred North Whitehead, *Religion in the Making* (Cleveland: World Publishing, 1961), p. 16.

Chapter 8

1. Richard Dawkins, *The Selfish Gene* (New York: Oxford University Press, 1976), p. 52.
2. Ernst Mayr, "Evolution," *Scientific American* 239 (1978), p. 52.
3. Francisco J. Ayala, "The Mechanisms of Evolution," *Scientific American* 239 (1978), p. 59.
4. Mayr, "Evolution," p. 52.
5. Mayr, "Evolution," p. 52.
6. U. Franke et al., "The Occurrence of New Mutants in the X-Linked Recessive Lesch-Nyhan Disease," *American Journal of Human Genetics* 28 (1976), pp. 123–137.
7. Schubert M. Ogden, "Evil and Belief in God: The Distinctive Relevance of a Process Theology," *The Perkins School of Theology Journal* 31 (1978), pp. 29–34.
8. Alexander Pope, "Essay on Man," Epistle 1, *Selected Works of Alexander Pope*, edited by Louis Kronenberger (New York: Random House, 1951), p. 106.
9. Ogden, "Evil and Belief in God," p. 32.
10. Ogden, "Evil and Belief in God," p. 33.
11. David Ray Griffin, *God, Power, and Evil: A Process Theodicy* (Philadelphia: The Westminster Press, 1976), p. 251f.
12. Griffin, *God, Power, and Evil*, p. 269.

Chapter 9

1. Schubert M. Ogden, *Faith and Freedom* (Nashville: Abingdon Press, 1979), p. 77.
2. Richard Dawkins, *The Selfish Gene* (New York: Oxford University Press, 1976), p. 24.
3. Ernst Mayr, "Evolution," *Scientific American* 239 (1978), p. 50.
4. Stephen Jay Gould, *Ever Since Darwin* (New York: W. W. Norton, 1977); *The Panda's Thumb* (New York: W. W. Norton, 1980).
5. Gould, *Ever Since Darwin*, pp. 56–62.
6. Theodosius Dobzhansky, *The Biology of Ultimate Concern* (New York: New American Library, Meridian Books, 1969), pp. 32–33.
7. Gould, *The Panda's Thumb*, p. 190.
8. David Griffin, *God, Power, and Evil: A Process Theodicy* (Philadelphia: The Westminster Press, 1976), pp. 282–285.
9. Griffin, *God, Power, and Evil*, p. 284.
10. Richard C. Lewontin, "Adaptation," *Scientific American* 239 (1978) pp. 215–216.
11. Council on Environmental Quality and the Department of State, *The Global 2000 Report to the President. Entering the Twenty-First Century*, vol. 1 (Washington, D.C.: U.S. Government Printing Office, 1980), p. 37.
12. Griffin, *God, Power, and Evil*, p. 284.
13. Griffin, *God, Power, and Evil*, p. 284.
14. Conrad H. Waddington, *Biology, Purpose and Ethics* (Clark University Press, with Barre Publishers, 1971), pp. 44–51.
15. Ogden, *Faith and Freedom*, p. 90.
16. Ogden, *Faith and Freedom*, p. 82.
17. Maxine Singer, "Recombinant DNA Revisited," *Science* 209 (1980), p. 1318.

Index